DEAR PSYCHOSIS,

A STORY OF HOPE AND LOVE THROUGH
A FAMILY'S JOURNEY OF MENTAL HEALTH

Sarah Martin

with contributions from
Alice Martin & Jesse Martin

Published by Sarah Martin

Copyright © Sarah Martin 2022

All rights reserved. Except as permitted under the *Copyright Act 1968*, (for example, a fair dealing for the purposes of study, research, criticism or review) no part of this book may be reproduced, stored in a retrieval system, or transmitted in any form or by any means without prior written permission from Sarah Martin. For further information, see sarahmartinauthor.com

Every effort has been made to trace and acknowledge copyright. However, should any infringement have occurred the publishers tender their apologies and invite copyright owners to contact them.

Cover design by Rebecca Hugonnet

Cover photograph by Alice Martin

Edited by Lu Sexton and Stephanie Preston

Printed by Ingram Spark

Martin, Sarah

Dear Psychosis,

ISBN print 978-0-6456449-1-3

ISBN ebook 978-0-6456449-9-9

Disclaimer

The material in this publication is of the nature of general comment only and does not represent professional advice. It is not intended to provide specific guidance for any particular circumstances and it should not be relied upon for any decision to take action or not to take action on any matter which it covers. Readers should obtain professional advice where appropriate, before making any such decision. To the maximum extent permitted by law, the author and publisher disclaim all responsibility and liability to any person, arising directly or indirectly from any person taking or not taking action based on the information in this book.

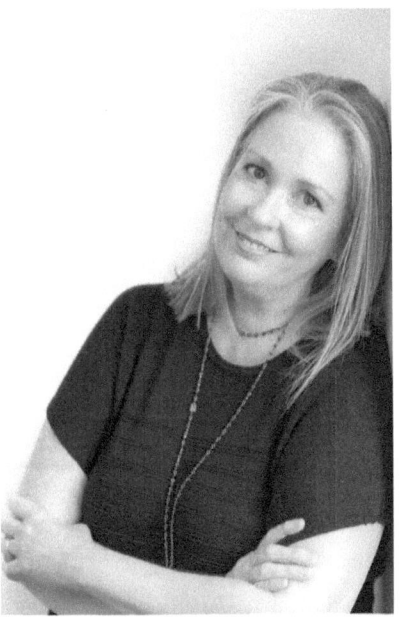

Sarah Martin is wife to Shane and mother to three beautiful but very different adult children, two cats, and a dog who thinks she's human.

Despite being an experienced theatre nurse and part of an extended family of medical professionals, nothing could have prepared Sarah for navigating the health system after her daughter Alice began experiencing psychosis and later, bipolar disorder.

Dear Psychosis, is Sarah's first book and describes not only the dramatic rescue of her unwell daughter from Turkey, but the ongoing impact of helping a loved one deal with mental illness.

Most of all, it is a story of recovery, hope and the power of family.

When not tackling the stigma and silence around mental illness, Sarah loves playing golf and making and baking sourdough bread.

*To my husband Shane, with his never-ending support!
My sons, Jesse who kept us grounded and Harry who showed us
the strength and resilience of a young adult.*

*To my amazing daughter Alice, without her courage, strength
and determination, this book would not
have been written.*

Dear Psychosis,

I have seen the darkness.

I have felt the anger.

I have touched the sadness.

I have grieved what was lost.

I have cried over the unfairness.

I have succumbed to the silence.

I will not speak.

I have welcomed the light amidst the darkness.

I have found strength through the anger.

I have embraced the sadness.

I have shouted my grief to the heavens.

I have wiped the tears away.

I will speak.

I am strong.

I am proud.

I am ready to share.

I. Am. Breaking. The. Silence.

By Sarah Martin

Contents

Preface — xiii
Introduction — 1

1. Facebook friend request — 4
2. Sunday — 20
3. Before — 22
4. Destination Istanbul — 25
5. Exposure to Captagon — 32
6. Landed in Istanbul — 43
7. Flashback: Suma Beach — 49
8. Downtown Istanbul — 57
9. Flashback: the kitten — 60
10. Impressions of Alice — 65
11. Flashback: trouble in Istanbul — 78
12. Mum and Jesse in the Bull — 86
13. Flashback — 98
14. Last day in the Bull — 100
15. Airport chaos — 106
16. Home — 115
17. Doctors, doctors, doctors — 120
18. White walls — 125
19. Father's Day — 130
20. Back home — 136

21. USpace	155
22. Out for lunch	167
23. Flashback: Krka National Park	171
24. A gift	173
25. Alice comes home	176
26. Friends	186
27. Turning point	190
28. Study	193
29. Houssain	200
30. Saviours	203
31. The future	205
Epilogue	212
Acknowledgements	222
Further resources	226

Psychosis, the dictionary says, is:

A severe mental disorder, with or without organic damage, which may be chronic or transient, characterised by derangement of personality and loss of contact with reality, causing a deterioration of normal social functioning.

Preface

What happens when you can't protect your children from something that is so hidden that no one can see it?

In 2015, our daughter Alice had her first episode of psychosis.

The rug was pulled out from under our feet and the blindfold ripped unceremoniously from our eyes when mental ill health was flung at our front door. We didn't ask for it to come inside, but it did.

It sat at our table uninvited and unwelcome.

We would come to imagine this Dear Psychosis as tentacles slowly wrapping themselves around our daughter, and sometimes around us too.

Why her? Why Alice? Why?

The answer was we had no idea.

When our children turn a certain age, we realise that they need to spread their wings, fly and broaden their horizons. Sometimes they fail and pick themselves up, dust themselves off and get on with it, and occasionally they don't. I wonder if it is how we deal with these moments that ultimately shapes their life?

When the mental health train struck, we became silent in our grief. Of what we as a family had lost, but most importantly grieving that Alice herself was slowly disappearing.

We were going in oblivious, with no clue as to what was ahead.

It didn't take long to be envious of friends and families that seemed to have it all. The beautiful, perfect families. Even if they had flaws, they were still perfect in my eyes.

On the few occasions we went out in that first year, Shane and I remained silent about the battles we were fighting at home. Dealing with it together, with a psychiatrist, a psychologist, and a concoction of drugs to keep Alice well.

No one knew.

No one knew or could help us because we were scared to share, for fear of Alice being judged. In my mind the life that I had mapped out for her was over.

Her brain was shut down and the strangeness had started.

She had voices in her head.

Conspiracy theories abounded.

The television was listening in to us.

She thought she had been implanted with a microchip in Istanbul and that it was still in her.

She could not read or write.

She could not draw in those adult colouring-in books, and certainly in those early days she could not have a conversation without it being completely delusional.

These delusions led to tricky conversations. You might not realise until halfway through it, that you weren't actually having the conversation with her that you thought you were. It was often hard to define things she said as fact or fiction, or the two would be jumbled together. We could sometimes find the essence but, in all honesty, we would give up after a while and would try and divert the conversation or mindset.

I would say, "I don't understand what you are talking about, can you explain again?" Often followed up with, "Let's go outside for a walk or cup of tea."

That simple chat you thought you were having, never, ever, really existed.

The diversion would either be met with indifference or anger.

When she became angry, she would throw verbal grenades at us. This could go on for a few minutes or become a rant that lasted for quite a while.

When these verbal grenades came our way, I could not see the light at the end of the tunnel. In fact, my only vision was of her having no life at all.

In those moments, I often could not stomach it, and would tell her she needed to stop talking as we were going nowhere. Inside, my heart was breaking for her and for all of us.

The sadness I felt was often intense and overwhelming.

Still, Shane and I essentially kept silent about what was happening at home. Too scared to share our story, our grief, and our heartbreak for what the future might be. It looked so very bleak.

But.

Spoiler alert – this story does have a positive ending.

We needed good healthcare, the perfect psychiatrist and psychologist for Alice, medications, house rules and routine, routine, routine.

It may not be what I envisioned for us as a family when we

started having children, but to be blatantly honest, none of our kids fit the mould. They all march to the beat of their own drum and have always thought outside the square. They would never have walked a straight line regardless of what we did.

So, what led me to writing a book? A narrative non-fiction book at that!

It started out as a cathartic bout of writing for me, a mother whose daughter was lost within the unexpected consequences of mental health, psychosis, bipolar, anxiety and depression, with often only my husband to talk to.

On any given day, I could be a nurse first and a mother or wife last, that's just the way it is, isn't it? As we grow up, our roles change depending on who or what needs us the most.

Like many others that have gone before us, and sadly to those who are coming after us, we needed the gift of hope.

Writing ended up being my therapy. An outlet where I could voice, without burdening or, dare I say, worrying or boring the small number of family and friends we had shared our ever-so-secret secret with.

Expressing what was going on in our everyday life, uncensored and directly from the heart, soon became my mission and my passion.

I would be lying if I didn't say that the year after Alice's first psychosis was the hardest time I have ever had in more than fifty years of life. Emotionally I was blown around like a sunflower in the wind. Roots holding firm, but frightened that I would break with the weight I felt that I was carrying on my shoulders.

My words began to multiply. Six months after our return from Istanbul, it became clear that I had more than an article but not enough for a book.

I started to think that perhaps I, no, *we* could write and share our journey with families and caregivers going through something similar. Most importantly, I wanted these families to believe in hope and know they are not alone. On a broader scale, my wish is for healthcare workers, doctors and nurses read it, to look at the other side of the coin. To see what is really happening in the homes of their patients, and thus create positive change. To treat the whole family, and to share in the wisdom and knowledge of those of us who have been in darkness.

I asked Alice if she felt she could put pen to paper but it wasn't until a year after her return from Istanbul that Alice emailed me the words that she had written. To be honest, I was not expecting her to recall much, and if she did, I was doubtful that I would be able to add it to our book. What Alice gave me was an amazing insight into her psychosis. Her words are confronting, frightening, and fascinating. A no-holds-barred account of what she went through while in Istanbul and then back at home.

I then asked our oldest son, Jesse, who was studying medicine, to add his words. To recount the week that he spent with us at the most critical time in Istanbul. To add further crucial observations and insight, not only of Alice at that time, but of me too. Our writing then turned into page after page of our story and this book was born.

Mental illness is silent and often invisible, as people (and we were those people) are reluctant to 'out' themselves or their loved one due to perceived repercussions that sadly exist in our society today.

By reading or listening to us, you are not only helping break the silence on mental illness, but you are assisting us in making as much noise as possible.

This book is NOT a self-help book.

What it is, is a story. It is our story.

Why is it so important that it is told?

If we don't share our experience …

The silence. Will. Continue.

Introduction

The Grand Tour. Some would call it a rite of passage, a post-school ritual, an overseas adventure, or a well-trodden path taken by many young people, whether within their own country or further afield. In 2015 it was our daughter's turn. Her year for excitement and adventure. Her time to grow and experience the 'trip of a lifetime'.

Having finished her university studies, a Bachelor of Arts and Communication, in June 2015, our twenty-one-year-old daughter, Alice, travelled overseas for an adventure through Europe. In London she met up with her older brother Jesse, Jesse's girlfriend Ella and their friend, Micca, before heading off on a trip they called their 'Roads Less Travelled Tour'. They bought a cheap car in Madrid, then together spent six weeks travelling before Jesse and Ella headed home to Melbourne, Micca to Greece and Alice to Turkey.

Once in Turkey Alice checked into a youth hostel near Taksim Square, the tourist quarter of Istanbul, where she met and hung out with a melting pot of wonderful humans from all over the world, seeking adventure, hope and freedom. She met a Syrian guy, who worked at the youth hostel she was staying at and who introduced her to his friends. These friends were fellow Syrians, displaced by the ravages of war from their homeland, and who were now living in Istanbul waiting for their next chapter.

They embraced Alice immediately and loved her simply for being her.

These were the people that would ultimately save Alice's life.

Istanbul, August 2015

She is running down the street, hair flying wildly around her face. Her head searches frantically from side to side, looking for something, anything. Her eyes are filled with fear and her throat has closed so much that no words can escape. Her arms are waving like windmills in a gale. A car stops beside her, and she wrenches the door open. Someone grabs her from behind and pulls her back. She lashes out at them. Trying to push them away, punching and hitting whoever has trapped her and suddenly it's like she's moving in slow motion.

Her world goes black.

CHAPTER 1

Facebook friend request

Saturday 29 August 2015

Sarah

The day was ushered in by one of those glorious sun-filled winter mornings where you would rather stay at home than go to work or a conference on your day off. But there I was sitting in a room filled with nurses at the National Day Surgery Conference, earning "continuing education points" required to maintain my nurse's registration. The seminar was called, ironically, 'Wellness for Life'.

I was a registered nurse, and had worked in the operating theatres for what seemed to be the last fifty years … actually, that isn't too far off the mark.

A few lectures in and I was trying hard not to yawn in the dimly lit auditorium. A huge curtain obliterated an enormous window and stopped the beautiful sunlight entering. A speaker stepped onto the stage and up to the podium, a very pregnant young woman. She began by saying that this was the second time that she'd given a speech about depression and asked us to pardon her nerves. Plastic rows of seats supported nurses with varying degrees of interest, engagement, and wakefulness. There is no adrenaline in the room, except perhaps for the speaker chancing her hand.

I nodded my head in support as she commenced her speech with a simple statement: "Depression can happen to anyone."

I thought about how it has no borders and does not care how much money you have, how educated you are or what job you do. Mental illness does not care what side of the fence you sit on.

During her speech, I glanced at my mobile phone. There was a Facebook request from someone who I thought might be a friend of my twenty-one-year-old daughter, Alice, who was traveling alone overseas.

Scammer, I thought before turning my attention back to the speaker who outlined her ongoing struggle and bravery in dealing with depression and postnatal depression. She finished to a standing ovation.

The next speaker started talking about laparoscopic banding surgery or gastric bypass surgery. He was only a few minutes into his presentation and my eyes joined the dozens of others glazing over. I looked at my trusty phone to occupy myself and this time there was an iMessage from the same name that had come up an hour before on the Facebook friend request.

I did not then know why but my heart started to beat a bit

quicker. I immediately recalled my shock a few days earlier when I had seen photographs of Alice with thick black marker pen all over her beautiful face.

I had waited for Alice to reply to my WhatsApp text in response to the image, hopefully saying that all was good.

There was no one to call, no one.

So, I waited and waited.

Finally, the day after the message with the image of her face covered in graffiti she had replied, "Ta-da", with a picture of her clean face.

Then, in that lecture, my mother's instinct was going off like a siren in my head, alarming. With shaking hands and ice-cold fingers, I opened the message from this person, this stranger.

11:07 am

Hey Sarah,
My name is Houssain.
I am a friend of Alice's in Istanbul.
I need to talk to you about Alice.
I know there is a big time difference between Istanbul and Sydney so I won't sleep, I will wait for you to get online and have some time to reply.

My fingers shook as I wrote: *Hi, I'm here.*

Immediately he replied.

Ah, thank God, Sarah. I'm worried about your Alice.

My heart started pounding.

My hands shook.

I needed to get out.

I whispered to Pip, my nursing colleague, 'Just going out for a minute.'

Houssain: *She's been wired for a while now. I cannot be sure, but I think she is showing signs of a major depression or schizophrenia.*

My brain exploded.

Wait! What?

This came from nowhere! Or had it … In some ways it was like pieces of a puzzle were finally coming together.

My daughter is in Istanbul. She is suffering and I'm not there.

My hands were shaking uncontrollably, my heart still pounding, and my eyes filled with tears. As I walked out of the lecture hall and past a table, I picked up some napkins, took a deep breath, wiped a stray tear that had snuck from my eye and told myself to get a grip.

I walked around the large, soulless tea-break area, looking lost and no doubt confused. I needed to find somewhere quiet, where I could be invisible.

I messaged back, Can I ring you?

Houssain sent me his number, but it didn't connect when I dialled it.

Neither did my husband's mobile phone when I tried over and over to reach him. He and our younger son Harry were playing golf. He would have turned his phone to silent. I left a text asking him to call me.

I felt desperate.

Again, I tried the Istanbul number, over and over. As much as I wanted to, I could not make it connect.

Houssain then sent me his friend's number, but that didn't work either.

My heart kept racing.

Why won't this work! My frustration was growing.

I needed to contact this man and I did not know how.

Think, think, what can I do to solve this problem?

I rang my twenty-four-year-old son Jesse, who lives in Melbourne studying medicine. I thought, *He will know what to do.*

It's Saturday morning and I knew he had been out for a big night of drinking and partying. Nonetheless. I rang.

Pick up the phone, Jess.

He didn't answer.

I hung up. Took a breath. The panic I felt was nearly overwhelming me. Focus, focus and try Jesse again.

His sleep-filled voice finally answered, and he heard me crying down the phone, panic-stricken.

Dragging in a deep gulping breath, I managed to speak, somewhat incoherently, something about Alice.

Then I broke down and sobbed. Not the loud emotional crying but the sort where your shoulders shake and you find it hard to breathe.

Jesse couldn't get any sense out of me for a few minutes. *What must he think?*

BREATHE.

Jess said he would contact this man in Istanbul. I would need to wait.

Jesse

Sometime before 11 am I received a phone call from Mum. I screened the first call. Saturday mornings in my final year doing a Bachelor of Medicine at Monash University in Melbourne weren't really for talking ... But the phone immediately rang again. A double dial usually means something is time critical. Last time it happened she was at the post office sending me a package but had forgotten my address. Probably something similar, I thought.

I didn't want to miss out on a care package, so I picked up the phone and swiped right.

Instantly, I knew that something was very wrong. What exactly, I had absolutely no clue. I could barely make out what she was saying through the combination of tears and incomprehensible noises coming from the other end of the line. I sat up in bed and forced myself to wake up in that moment. My girlfriend, Ella, was now awake and worried at what she was hearing. I raised my hands in the air and whispered, "No idea what's going on, Mum's crying!'

I let Mum go for a few more seconds but quickly realised her panic on the other end of the line was not going to allow my own comprehension of whatever was happening. "Hold on, Mum, slow down. I'm here. Take a few deep breaths and when you're ready tell me what's happened?" I managed to intercept and slow things down enough to start a conversation. My own heart rate had increased significantly.

Over the rest of the call, Mum was able to recount what had transpired in the last thirty minutes before she'd rung me in her state of panic and fear.

I had the contact number and immediately dialled Turkey. The dial tone lasted a few seconds before it broke away, replaced by an exhausted, "Hello."

Houssain began to tell me about Alice's recent behaviour changes and that he was worried for her safety and for his own. She had hardly slept in the last week and she was prone to impulsivity and she had these startling thoughts of grandeur that were often tinged with paranoia.

I was concerned but I'm not sure that the seriousness of Alice's mental health had quite hit me. It was a difficult conversation to have with another person, but an even more difficult one to have with myself. The natural human tendency is to hope for the best, especially when the worst is something that you want to avoid. Houssain told me what was happening, and it was up to me to decide what all of it meant. Over the coming days, with more information and more time, the hope would slowly slip away to be replaced by an immutable reality.

I had fortunately just finished my mental health semester at university so I was at least armed with questions I could ask Alice and Houssain. After speaking to Houssain for some time, we ended the call so I could talk to Alice.

She answered the phone calmly, in an ethereal manner. There was a tranquillity in her voice that shrouded the mess of thoughts that must have been going on inside. Initially this put me at ease. Alice's affect through the phoneline combined with what was likely copious denial on my end. After the platitudes were said, I went straight to conducting a mental health risk assessment. I directly asked whether she had any feelings of self-harm, suicidal intentions, suicidal plans, homicidal intentions, homicidal plans, as well as questions about financial and sexual risk taking. The aim was to have Alice's personal safety guaranteed in the context of her own ideation and intentions (as much as you can from a brief, initial conversation like this).

Alice wasn't having intrusive thoughts of suicide or self-harm, or of harm to others or any urges for potentially unsafe risk taking. This was reassuring, but did I believe what she had said? The concerning content was the tangential and at times derailed thinking that was revealed in her speech. Paranoid ideas, delusions and what sounded like auditory and visual hallucinations. I would need to check in with Houssain and the rest of the housemates to confirm.

How much faith can you have in a risk assessment from a potentially psychotic individual? Did I even think Alice could be psychotic at that time, or did I want to believe that she was just being Alice?

I carried on the phone call hoping to gain more insight into Alice's thought process, but also to just have a normal conversation with Alice, like to see how her trip had been since I last spoke to her.

It is interesting for me to look back on the start of this journey, to see with perfect hindsight what was happening. I recall at the time being quite confident after this conversation that Alice would be able to be put on a plane to London where we have some family who she could stay with until she either came home or could continue her travels. Houssain was adamant this was not an option. This was perhaps the most telling aspect about Alice's headspace.

How many people in your life would you have said were unsafe to get on a plane? Did I really believe it?

I hung up the phone and called Mum back to reassure her and let her know that it seemed to me that Alice was at low risk of immediate harm, with her friends nearby (though tired). I suggested that Mum call Alice to see what she thought and to gain a second opinion. My timeline around this period is somewhat skewed and, to be honest, I was hungover from the night before. A lot was happening almost simultaneously and even my own thoughts and opinions on the situation were changing just as fast and fluidly.

As with any evolving situation, new information came in fast and I was alerted to the odd text messages Alice had been sending Mum over the past few weeks, more history, more solid information, and the picture of declining mental health was certainly beginning to take form.

Sarah

Still Saturday.

I was outside the conference room, at the very end of the veranda, sitting on a hard white plastic chair. The wobbly table was one of those pseudo-fancy glass ones and I was attempting to be invisible. I could hear the clinking of coffee and teacups being set up for lunch when someone dropped a cup and it smashed splattering coffee and shards of glass all over the ground. I thought it sounded like me, shattering into a million pieces. I felt melodramatic and guilty that those feelings were building up and creeping out of me, when I didn't know exactly what was happening to Alice. I think the fear and panic of going through those first few hours overwhelmed me. I lost a bit of me that was eaten up by anxiety and in the panic of the moment.

I took a breath. I tried to clear my head of negativity. I searched the internet for phone codes now that I knew that someone else was helping me. I soon saw that I was so distressed that I had been using the incorrect country code for Turkey.

Jesse messaged me, *Got onto the guy. Call me, Mum.*

I tried Shane again, still nothing.

People just don't contact you from the other side of the world for nothing, do they?

When I finally got onto him, Houssain told me he had just left his apartment to talk outside and Alice is finally sleeping after being awake for days. Her behaviour, according to Houssain, was extremely erratic and odd from what he had seen of her over the past four weeks.

Soon after, both Jess and I spoke with Alice, not for long but enough to know that all was not right.

She was quietly spoken.

She was flat.

She was rambling.

Was all this due to her simply being tired? It was early hours of the morning in Istanbul, I would be exhausted if someone rang and woke me in the middle of the night and I wouldn't sound sparky either. Was this guy overreacting to Alice's behaviour? Were we feeding off his anxiety?

So many questions that we needed answers to.

12:37 pm

It took over an hour in conversations going backwards and forwards between Jesse, Houssain and me to get some semblance of clarity.

Back at the conference lunch area, I closed my eyes to focus and think but all I could hear was the steady chatter of staff sorting out the buffet table for lunch, others laughing and every now and then a phone ringing.

No one noticed the forlorn person in their midst and for that I was grateful.

My concerned work colleague came to find me at lunchtime. She could immediately see that something wasn't right at all. My eyes were puffy and tinged with red, and my nose probably rivalled Rudolph's. My hand clenched a random napkin that I'd been using to wipe away the tears. I was relieved to see her and I recounted what had happened, with that tear-soaked serviette scrunched in one hand and her hand holding my other. I was trying not to cry. Fortunately for me, my colleague was extremely level-headed and kept me grounded for the next hour. I was so appreciative to get another perspective from someone sitting beside me who I could touch and feel.

The immediate problem was that I feared for Alice's wellbeing and there was no plan in place yet.

Jesse was in Melbourne.

Shane was still uncontactable.

Continuing from our last text message, Jesse had been busy thinking of what we could or should do. At this stage we were wondering if Alice could fly to London.

I looked at my phone and the time stared back at me. Surprisingly, it was only two and a half hours since receiving Houssain's first message. Time was dragging.

I stayed on at the conference.

Leaving would have meant going home to an empty house with my racing thoughts and increasing anxiety over Alice's wellbeing.

There was nothing I could do at that stage. My heart was breaking and there was the overwhelming uncertainty as to what was happening to Alice.

It was four hours after I first tried to contact Shane that he finally returned my call and I couldn't pick up my phone fast enough.

I started with the usual, "Everything is okay but …" My voice was wobbly as I spoke quietly to him, eyes focused on the outside world, watching everyday life continuing to unfold around me.

Shane was shocked, although he knew something was up due to the number of missed calls from me. After I filled him in, I asked him to call Jesse, so I could make my way home. I suddenly had an urgent desire to get home and be around those I love.

Meanwhile, I had shared our thoughts with Houssain about getting Alice on a plane to London and this was met with a resounding NO. "*She cannot fly to London, she cannot fly by herself, she cannot BE by herself.*"

If I was worried before, my concerns increased tenfold. What did he mean, *she cannot BE by herself?*

On my drive home, I turned the radio up and put the window down to let the fresh air hopefully blow my spinning thoughts out of my brain and rid them from the car.

Focus, I thought, *just get home.*

I walked up the pathway with a heavy heart and a sadness about what might be happening. With tears filling my eyes, I opened our front door to Shane's immediate embrace and cried quietly on his shoulder. We stayed this way for a while. Both wiping away our tears when we let go.

It surprised me that the day was still beautiful, no storm was brewing, the sun was shining and shockingly, the sky had not fallen in.

Life went on around us.

Shane and I discussed at length if it was some sort of international scam, and if Alice could have been in danger somehow, or if the facts were exactly as we had been told.

What it all came down to was taking the word and observations of a man we had never met. Should we take the advice of a stranger? Did we trust a man we did not know? There was much discussion on this. Jesse and I had spoken with Houssain and our gut said that we believed him, although the entire scenario seemed bizarre.

The conversations we had with Alice were short. She seemed tired, softly spoken and at times confused, enough for us to be concerned. She herself could not put into words what was wrong with her. She seemed listless and uninterested in what we were talking about.

What we did know is that our guy, Houssain, had been in Istanbul for eighteen months. Houssain, Rima, Kholod, Ba Sim, Batool and Basook. These were the names we needed to remember.

Amongst these folk were an architect, an information technology worker, an actress, a music producer, a mum. All from Syria, displaced from their homeland. They were all struggling to get work to survive. Yet here they were apparently helping a girl from across the world through a crisis that no one expected.

They were our only link to our daughter.

What sealed the deal was reflecting on the strange text messages from Alice in the previous weeks. That photograph of her beautiful face marred with lines that she had drawn with a thick black marking pen.

Someone from Beyond Blue, a mental health helpline, was a guest speaker earlier that day at the conference. I had taken some pamphlets and, with the number fortunately at my fingertips, I decided to give them a call. I explained the situation to someone on the other end of the phone. I needed affirmation that we were doing the right thing.

"Yes, brilliant," he said. "But one last thing, here is the number of the Australian embassy in Istanbul, in case her health declines any further while you are in transit and she needs to be taken to hospital."

I had already spoken with Houssain regarding hospitalisation and medical treatment. He was adamant that Istanbul was not the place to take her to hospital for a mental health matter. English is not spoken widely in Turkey and he was concerned that Alice's medical needs would get lost in translation. He was of the opinion that while she had familiar faces around her, she would be safe.

From the other side of the planet the only thing we could do was believe him.

The decision was made that we needed to get there to assess the true situation as soon as possible. We had a family discussion that included our thirteen-year-old son, Harry. We didn't want to have whispered conversations around him when something was so clearly going on. We made sure he understood everything we talked about, although I was doubtful of how much he absorbed or understood. The important objective for us was that we were a team, a family unit that would fight this fight united.

There were two certainties, Shane needed to stay home and work, and I needed to go. The one major fly in the ointment was that I'm a hopeless traveller. I suffer terrible motion sickness to the degree that I get nauseous on a ski lift. I will not go on boats and even a blow-up air mattress floating on water is out of the question. Therefore, I do not take too well to flying. I had never flown internationally by myself, not that it was an insurmountable problem, but was a sticking point for my already anxious self. Jesse declared he could take a few days off his university studies. He was between subjects and had the week off but would only come if I thought I would need him, as cost was a huge factor. Thankfully we decided Jess should come. It was the best decision we made.

Our flights were booked on Qatar Airways, leaving Melbourne the following night. We would worry about the money later. Turkish visas were purchased online, and accommodation was researched, but not found. We wanted a hotel close to Houssain and his friends, but we would leave that in Shane's capable hands, and he would sort it out while we are in the air.

Jesse

It's interesting to see to what degree we as a family may have been denying the severity of the information that we had been given.

Or if perhaps the seriousness of Alice's behaviour had not quite been delivered as forcefully as needed, and whether we'd stumbled over language barriers, the inherent taboo of mental health and a propensity for mental illness to be played down. This all combined with our own denial – a sort of 'Alice will be alright' mindset – to affect how serious we thought the situation actually was. But it was when we were told that Alice was not going to be safe enough to fly alone that we truly realised the possible extent of Alice's mental health crisis.

Not safe enough to fly.

CHAPTER 2

Sunday

Sunday 30 August 2015

Sarah

I slept terribly that night, waking up about every hour, continually checking the clock and my phone to see if Alice or Houssain had tried to message me. The night was interminable and when dawn finally arrived, I fell into an exhausted sleep.

We spent the day running round trying to find my anti-nausea motion sickness medication, packing, adding a few pieces of clothing for Alice, and lastly ringing my parents and my sister to let them know what was happening. I held my emotions together until my parents, without question or judgement, offered to pay for our plane tickets and wished us a safe and uneventful return home. They had no idea how much they had relieved us of a huge financial burden. Tears flowed.

Shane decided he would call his sister and then my brothers when Jesse and I got to Istanbul. My brothers are doctors, married to doctors, and need black-and-white information which we clearly did not have. We certainly had a lot of mud to wade through to get to the clear stuff. So, in the first instance the information Shane gave them was vague at best because, at that moment, we really had no idea what exactly was wrong with Alice. We would not put a label on it to anyone, even my family.

By now it was a little over twenty-four hours since receiving the news that Alice needed help.

Shane and Harry dropped me at the airport. I felt like an emotional wrecking ball had hit me, but I had time to get myself together before I reached Melbourne and met Nearly-doctor Jesse at the international airport. We departed a few hours later at 11 pm.

We may have left Shane, Harry and Jesse's girlfriend, Ella, behind but they were with us in spirit. Flying into the unknown.

We had already discussed every scenario we could think of; the good, the bad and the ugly.

What IF she was unfit to travel?

What IF she deteriorated further before we got there?

What IF she was perfectly fine?

What IF it was a scam?

We had no idea what awaited us in Istanbul, we were relying on the observations of a man we knew nothing about but had to trust. The safety of our girl was completely in his hands.

CHAPTER 3

Before

May to July 2015

Alice

Our Roads Less Travelled journey had started in London. When I arrived from Australia, Jesse, Ella and Micca had sorted out our travel itinerary and I was just happy to tag along and go with the flow. So, it was a fait accompli that our first stop was in Spain, more specifically Madrid.

Here Jesse and Micca travelled out to the industrial area about forty-five minutes outside of central Madrid to hopefully buy a car. They took it for a test drive, it seemed okay and so they began the bartering process. Only thing was, the dealership didn't have any English speakers, and neither of the boys could speak Spanish!

Technology saved the day! Google Translate was used with one sentence written at a time, then the computer screen turned to face the other side of the bartering table. Over twenty minutes a deal was made and they shook hands to trade seven hundred euros for the 1996 Ford Mondeo (Ghia edition).

It had a sunroof that did not open, fake mahogany on all the trimmings, doors that creaked when you opened them and 250,000 kilometres on the clock, but it drove and it didn't rattle. Jesse and Micca drove the car back to Ella and me in the city, where we were able to meet 'Scummy' for the first time. The name for the car came after we listened to an Artic Monkeys song called 'When the Sun Goes Down'. In the song they sing about a scummy man who drives a Ford Mondeo. The name fit, so Scummy it was called!

So, on a wing and a prayer, with music blaring, we started on our travels. Four jubilant Euro-trippers squeezed into a little sedan with all our backpacks in the boot.

Most of our trip was carefree and fun. We would spend our days relaxing on the beach, drinking, eating, sleeping and walking through towns. Put this on repeat and that was our daily routine in a nutshell.

***

Monday 20 July 2015

The first night in Istanbul, I was with friends I had met in Bulgaria: Abbey, Nate and Edwin. We were on our way to find something to eat when Nate stumbled across an artist's studio and ushered us inside. The artist's name was Avni, he was around seventy years old. He was short, about five foot five, with greying hair and a compulsive addiction to smoking large cigarettes rolled out of paper with little crowns on them.

We ended up staying at Avni's studio, which had wall-to-wall paintings, some leaning on the wall four-deep. There was a table littered with paint brushes, scattered with years of paint, jars of turpentine and the smell to go with it. The chairs were rickety and probably nearly as old as Avni himself. We were there with Anvi's nephew, who could speak a smattering of English, till the early hours of the morning, just drinking and smoking Turkish cigarettes. We left feeling energised and ready to sleep comfortably. This experience amazed me and reinforced my desire to spend a couple of weeks getting lost in Istanbul.

A couple of days later, Manar, a Syrian guy who worked at the hostel, invited us to have tea at his apartment. I remember feeling very sick with a sore throat and runny nose, but I had a strong Fear Of Missing Out, so I went.

Despite the sickness, I remember feeling free and light walking the streets to Manar's. We had tea when we arrived. Here I met Ashraf and soon after in walked Houssain, the other roommate.

Little did I know then that that was where I would be spending the next month.

CHAPTER 4

Destination Istanbul

Sunday 30 August 2015

Jesse

I met Mum at the check-in gate at Melbourne Airport. She gave me a grin that might have been a grimace and a hug that trembled with uncertainty. While waiting for the flight, we discussed the possible scenarios that might unfold once we landed in Istanbul. The scenario we both liked the most was the one in which Alice was ill, but not so ill that the holiday couldn't continue with Mum by her side in London to browse the old museums and galleries before they both returned home. I guess red flags just look like flags when you're wearing rose-coloured glasses. The scenario we liked the least was the one in which Alice was so sick that we would need to immediately book a return flight home to Australia.

The flight was going to be a solid day of blank time, in that we had no idea of any evolving situation on the ground and, really, even if we did there was no way we could speed up anything or change the course of any outcome until we landed and were face-to-face with Alice. The advantage to this was that I could hit the medical books and begin to form the initial body of evidence that would eventually aid in the diagnosis of whatever was going on inside Alice's mind.

I had recently completed a psychiatry term at university and additionally had the golden book of mental health diseases, *The Diagnostic and Statistical Manual of Mental Disorders* (the DSM-5), which had been updated only months before.

What I knew about Alice's behaviour could fit into a few diagnoses, such as schizophrenia (which often presents in those entering adulthood, like Alice), bipolar affective disorder and a major depressive episode with psychotic features. I read much of the DSM-5, but in my mind, I knew I had to be careful in that my role here would be mainly to get as much information as possible from Alice's friends, while taking down my own observations of her behaviour, thoughts, and speech when we arrived. I would be the conduit for the specialist to make a working diagnosis and give Alice the best chance for timely and correct treatment if she needed it.

Having said that, long haul flights are tedious at the best of times, so there was only so much I could do before losing attention. Many thanks to whomever decided to put three seasons of the slapstick, mindless but hilarious comedy *Brooklyn 99* on the plane entertainment system.

Sarah

As we sat in the aircraft at Melbourne airport preparing to depart, we could see the scenario a few ways. One was that this was a scam, or perhaps something more sinister, and we were flying into danger. The other, of course, was that Alice was ill and needed help. Meanwhile, the jets' voices rose to a full roar and we sped down the runway. To what?

Here I had plenty of time to think back over the past few years. I buckled my seatbelt, put my headphones on, closed my eyes and went back over events to see if I could find some clues. I know now in hindsight that some things were glaringly obvious.

It came as no surprise when in the final year of her degree Alice began to talk about heading overseas to travel for six months before finding a job. Over the last three years while at university, she had volunteered at a local public school teaching ethics to first graders, looked after a little girl three days a week after school and spent another couple of days where she worked at the local bottle shop, all to pay for her trip.

Like most mothers, my mind and heart were divided over what this holiday break meant. My girl was going away, and I knew I would miss her, but I also knew what a great opportunity it was and how much Alice would grow.

One day we have babies and it seems the next they are all grown up and it is their time to become an adult and experience life outside of the protective hub we make as a family.

So, it was with an excited but nervous heart I drove her out to the airport and sent her off. I tried not to cry at the departure gate but failed miserably.

So much had changed in the thirty-five years since I went on my first overseas holiday. Thank goodness for social media, as that would be our vision into her world while she was away.

Jess and Ella returned home to Australia after six weeks travelling with Alice. Micca had gone to Greece and Alice said she was keen to have some down time, to write in her journal, relax and breathe, before heading to Turkey.

Shortly after arriving in Istanbul, Manar, one of the Syrian workers employed at the hostel where Alice was staying, took her and a few other travellers on a brief tour of the city and introduced them to his friends. Through him, she met a young man, Houssain, who we noted had made an appearance on social media, plus she talked about him in text messages. So, to us it looked like they were becoming close. A holiday romance it seemed was blossoming.

Alice organised a dinner where everyone that was staying in the hostel prepared a meal from their own culture and country. There were dishes from all around the world and those that could not cook joined in on decorating and gathering ingredients. The festivities of the day went long into the night with someone's bongo drums coming out, singing, dancing, stories and much laughter. This seemed to set the theme for the following week. We could hear the happiness in her voice over the phone when we talked, and a sense of relief filled me that she was having such a wonderful experience.

Then at the end of July, we had over a week of silence.

I felt quite anxious about not hearing from her. On the other hand, I knew that she was her own person and on holidays, but she was also now travelling by herself. Finally, a text arrived saying that she and a group of her friends had gone to a music festival a few hours away. I mentally berated myself for worrying.

The next weeks for her seemed to be filled with meeting people, including Avni, a local Turkish artist in his mid-seventies, who took an immediate shine to Alice. I am not sure how they communicated with each other as Avni spoke no English and Alice spoke no Turkish. My WhatsApp banter with Alice at this time revolved a lot around Avni and whether he had ulterior motives, and my mother instincts were going off. I questioned Alice and she was most offended that I would even think such a thing and then she laughed at me when she described him. He was this little wizened old man, with a weathered face, who smoked Turkish cigarettes all day and loved a glass or three of the local liquor. Alice adored him.

Around the middle of August Alice's text messages became a little 'strange' and disjointed and I brought them up with Shane, but he said, "Let her be, she is twenty-one and living the dream."

So I did.

***

A week earlier. Sydney

Alarm bells were beginning to sound in my brain but at this stage they were dull.

One afternoon, Alice and I were having a conversation via text and she sent me on a wild goose chase in our house looking for a rose quartz rock she had bought before she left on her travels. After about thirty minutes of looking, I finally found it.

Can you pick up the rose quartz for me, Mum?

This one? I send through a photograph.

Haha, no that's tiger eye.

This one?

It's the lump of pink that was by your bed for ages.

I post another photo of yet another rock

Wooooaaaa. That's Himalayan. Amethyst.

This one? I asked myself what the hell I was doing.

Yep, that's the one! Hehe thank you. You can have it haha.

Why did you need it?

I dunno, thanks.

Our conversation ended and I spent the next half hour trying to rationalise what just happened. I simply couldn't, so I pushed it aside and put my head in the sand, again.

Several days passed and I had just arrived at work at 5:50 in the morning when I noticed Alice had messaged me on WhatsApp. When I opened it, I lost my breath, my heart pounded and I had an instant headache. Alice had sent through a few photographs. I scrolled backwards and forwards through photos showing her with black marker drawn all over her beautiful face, like a thick black road map.

My heart beat out of my chest, and I texted her straightaway asking if everything was okay, then waited and waited for a reply.

The alarm bells really started exploding in my head.

I was so overwhelmed that I cried in the tiny sterile stock room in the hospital where all the instruments for surgery are kept. I was discovered there by one of my colleagues who tried valiantly to allay my fears. She hugged me and told me all was alright. I showed her the pictures and her eyes widened like saucers. She blinked a few times, not knowing what to say. I took a deep breath, rang Shane and sent him the photos. He had no words that could help me or himself.

There was nothing, NOTHING, to do but wait.

By the following week, my family's world was turned upside down and my son and I were on a plane winging our way on a 28,000 kilometre dash to bring our girl home.

***

Back in real time. Atatürk Airport, Istanbul

Finally, nearly twenty-four hours since we left Australia, we arrived in Istanbul, via Doha, at midday.

CHAPTER 5

Exposure to Captagon

26 July 2015

Alice

The first night with these guys in Istanbul, a bloke that my new friends knew offered me a pill of something I had never heard of before, Captagon (Fenethylline). The effects were described to me as uplifting and lively, just like coffee. Anyway, I swallowed my quarter of a pill, wondering what to expect from such a small amount.

I was speaking to my friend, Ashraf, he was telling me about the work he does with a humanitarian non-profit organisation, based in Syria. We also started to discuss the Syrian conflict, so we left the club and went for tea down the road. I was glued to this conversation; I had felt quite ignorant about the conflict and was keen to be educated.

At this stage I felt no different, but to be honest I was not giving my pill taking much thought.

By the time we got back to the club everyone had left already, so we walked back to the apartment together. When we got there, I felt quiet and reflective. I wrote a poem in my haste to make the most of the introverted mood. It was like my brain was stuck in fast-paced thoughts that needed to be smoothed out and blown around, like when kids blow bubbles from a wand. I re-read the poem to myself and added in some satirical lines. I thought I had written a masterpiece. I felt compelled to share it with the others in the room.

Without you

A storm seems elusive

Lost in time Space

Beats exclusive

Solo, times four, the countdown goes

And hum

Booms and beats

What is drum, in heart, senza eye – meets & chill, forever, &

bleed ... Together.

A third of what's necessary isn't really there in the eyes of plenty.

Forever hastening to make more of many ... Barely there.

A faded beat, familiar.

A third of a word, familiar. Fa- mi- ly - ha!

A. heard A. herd.

Misconception in ecstatic mention of splitting thirds, money turds. Oh shit.

Crashing words between worlds. What?

Like a dog without a bone. Ruff ruff

Anchor into the eyes, we will surf the nation's demise despite the grey skies (? Absurd!)

The sea is red with the blood of our brothers' sisters' mothers' cries. Fuck – and lives – dear father, we preach to you!! Our governmental brother?!

Step in, inside the beat <here> shut the fuck up – rakkia!

In our lineage, in our language we beseech for you to clear the floors

beneath the clouded plenty and let the blood of your once familiar

nation (see how fucked up that sounds) be lit!

Set fire to the dead leaves and let the roots migrate with make

believe manure under our feet.

Now I can hear how heavily the poem was influenced by Captagon. Anyway, I read it aloud and my friends really enjoyed it.
"*Did you write that just now?*"
"*Yes, I did.*"
Later I was sitting on the balcony alone and Kholod came out and said she thinks I am a genius.
It got to the point, so quickly, that when I entered rooms by myself it was like I was taken over, but it was so subtle at the start, and I guess I just tried to ignore the fact that something was deeply wrong. This was quite out of character for me. I wonder if this was shortly after I wrote in my journal, *Woke up this morning feeling flat for the first time in weeks. Tried to ride the wave out.*

It marks when delusions began trickling in, which perhaps kept me from being able to talk about what was going on inside my head in a rational manner. I would come back from a trip to the bathroom and Houssain would ask me, "Are you still here?" I would get defensive, unwilling to say what a difficult time I had just experienced in the bathroom alone.

***

Saturday 30 August 2015

The day before Mum's arrival I remember hanging out with Kholod and dancing, feeling like my state of mind was contagious and worrying for her. All I could do was dance to avoid feeling these distressing thoughts, yet I knew I didn't like dancing all that much and it felt unnatural.

I was under the illusion that Houssain had been implanted with a device that could detect thoughts and feelings. This delusion grew with every phone call he would make. I believe the delusion originated from a week before, when I asked about his time in jail in Syria. I felt terribly guilty of being a bad listener, something that was so foreign to me as I have always loved hearing people's stories, but it felt like something had crawled into my brain and put me in such a state of drowsiness I forgot everything he said.

After this I believed he had become an undercover 'bad guy' because he must have been brainwashed in jail. I thought he had three phones to 'triangulate' and thus disperse the messages from

Turkish authorities, to conceal his evil plans of possible illegal activities. One phone was given to him by a American girl that was at the party on Suma, her indifference towards me struck me as borderline rude. I was yet to establish where the other phones were and who gave them to him.

I distrusted the phone situation.

Going to sleep that night was horrible. I believed I was in the cosmically charged arena of the Bull. I refused to sleep, believing that morning was not going to come. I shut the door to the balcony as I thought bombs might rain from the sky. Someone moved the single mattress by the door, I only found out after that they did this in case I was to get up and leave in the middle of the night. Kholod fell asleep sitting upright. Bassem went and lay in Ashraf's bed and Houssain stayed with me.

My friends were protecting me from myself, and I didn't know it.

At the time my delusions were telling me not to trust these people. I thought Bassem may have been selling my energy to the French and that Houssain, as well as everything else he was doing, was plotting my abduction. When everyone went to sleep, I felt sad because of what they were going to do to me. Some part of me was still acknowledging that the delusions were not taking hold of all my reality, just.

Meanwhile, I hadn't eaten or slept properly in days.

***

Sunday 31 August 2015

The morning that Mum and Jess arrived I was fraught with delusions. Dad used to be in the navy, and he has friends who are still in it. I thought they knew I needed help, and the plan was that I had to leave the apartment and get in any car, as the driver would be 'one of these friends' and they would know where to take me, to assist me. I thought this was a scary burden, to have do it by myself, but I had to try and ensure I was there at the airport without tipping off the drone in Houssain's body. This would mean Mum's plane would be bombed down or she would be shot after getting off it. The scariest thing was knowing how numb I was, and that I may not be able to do anything that could help them.

I woke up early and showered. I wanted to leave straight away but thought better of it. I raided the fridge for some cheese and tomato, knowing I had not been eating. By the time I had packed a very small bag with my passport and other necessary things Houssain had woken up. I did not know what to do. I can't imagine the look on my face, but it must have been full of shock and desperation. I knew I was very early as Mum's flight came in around lunch time.

I was filled with mistrust and confusion. The delusions had gripped me so quickly that I was weary and bewildered, all my energy was going towards a fantastical mind dragon burning memories of a once 'normal' time. I can only imagine the scars that have been left on my brain.

I remember later, in hospital in Australia, I wanted Houssain to design me a tower where I could imagine that my thoughts would disturb no one and I would be protected by the mind dragon, but I never voiced it. This desire to be alone was hard to shrug off through my recovery.

There I was, frozen at the apartment door, standing on the mattress that someone was sleeping on, with Houssain asking, "What are you doing, where are you going?"

"For a walk," I said.

Houssain reminded me that my mum was coming and asked if I was excited. The truth was I was emotionless, all I felt was a state of physiological anxiety. My response was probably far from the truth. Hindsight is a good thing and I wish I felt close enough to the people I was with to talk about the strong delusions that gripped me, but it was too real and powerfully scary.

I didn't even feel close enough to myself to admit I was delusional.

I am not sure how long we waited in the apartment before we left it to drive to the airport, but it seemed like forever and I was impatient to go, or at least get out of the apartment as I needed to meet the car.

For whatever reason – the comedown from Captagon, the lack of sleep, the business of Istanbul, the lack of food, the lack of fresh air and exercise – I felt trapped. Houssain was tired, too. To me this came across as something to be afraid of. Was he working in secret throughout his 'holiday' for evil forces? I worried he had been working on a secret project that involved me and I wasn't sure how. I 'knew' so badly I had to get away, that on the walk to the car the morning of my mum's arrival I resorted to physical danger and attempted to choke Houssain not once but twice.

It was a horrible feeling holding life in your hands like that. But that was the desperation I felt, that's what the voices suggested I do. I kept missing the suggestions of the voices to get into a car or cab or a van. So, I took it out on poor Houssain, who was just trying to be there for me. I was terrified of what I thought Houssain was, or at least what my mind thought he was.

When we went outside, I ran down the road, frantically trying to escape. I wasn't doing a very good job. I knew I could be running faster, and I was confused as to why I wasn't running as hard as I could. I went about fifty metres when a taxi came past, I must have called out or waved my hands about in the air as the driver stopped, I opened the door and was just getting in the car when Houssain pulled me out. Fortunately, at the same time as this commotion was happening, Bassem pulled up with Kholod in the car and that diverted my attention from one of fear and escape to bewilderment at what was going on.

While this was all happening, Houssain continued talking to me in the gentlest of voices, what he was saying, I cannot recall, but whatever it was, it was calming.

They all ushered me into the car like bodyguards shielding a VIP, or on the flipside a victim being kidnapped by her assailants, but my mind had now switched to unbelievable, terrifying fear.

That is when I sat on a bomb. It was constantly vibrating under my bottom in the car on the way to the airport. I think I thought it was somehow connected to Houssain's drone and I had to do my best to stay calm and not think about the elephant in the room: the issue of Houssain being a baddie.

Bassem parked the car, and I remember taking off my mum's necklace because I believed it was giving me supernatural powers of hearing voices and air control (my star sign is Aquarius, an air sign). The necklace was the Egyptian symbol for 'Sarah' that had been given to Mum by her brother over forty years ago. She had given it to me so that she would always be with me when I was away.

We were early so we went to watch the planes flying over our heads. This would have been fun if I was in a different state of mind.

I believed I had to do yoga and try to remain very calm for Mum's plane to land safely. In my mind, Houssain was still working with forces of darkness to try and bring the plane down.

He asked me what he could do to help me, and I told him to just tell me to keep it or take it. Clearly this was a personal joke of mine, because when he said it, I laughed and stretched my arms out in front of me with my hands opened to receive and 'took' the thought as truth and then I saw a van across the road unloading parcels near us and I started walked towards it, to get in it.

Houssain said, "What are you doing?"

And I replied, "You told me to take it so I'm taking the thought to the next level."

Fortunately, he was able to move me away from the van and divert my attention elsewhere, because the urge to get in the van and away from Houssain was strong.

We eventually moved to wait for Mum in the terminal. I was flanked by my friends on either side and one behind me.

I couldn't see a plane from 'Sydney' on the arrivals board, so I didn't think she was coming. I tried to walk away but Houssain said, "What are you doing? Your mother is nearly here."

Out of desperation and confusion, I sat on the floor amid a sea of people and Kholod sat down with me. I was so grateful. I remember hoping that my condition, whatever it was, wasn't contagious and wouldn't affect her.

CHAPTER 6

Landed in Istanbul

Monday 31 August 2015

Sarah

We landed at Atatürk Airport in Istanbul exhausted and apprehensive. The very first thing I did was take my phone off flight mode and could see that there was a message from Houssain. He said they'd be meeting us at the arrival area. They managed to get a car, something had happened in the hours before our arrival with Alice. She was ok but he thought it best to meet us at the airport.

I didn't think any more of the message, I was just grateful to be there and one step closer to seeing our girl. Istanbul is a bustling, historic city of more than 15 million people, but I only had thoughts for one person, Alice.

We made our way through the dreariness of customs, then went straight out to find Alice and her friends in the overcrowded arrivals hall. We scanned the many groups of people standing around, a thick bouillabaisse jampacked with travellers and families all waiting to reunite with their loved ones. Finally, out of the corner of my eye I saw a striking movement and turned to watch a group of people pushing their way through the crowd. I could see her, Alice, bracketed by three of her exhausted but fantastic new friends. Time then seemed to go in slow motion, like in a movie where everyone else around you blurs into insignificance and the people you are wanting to see take forever to get to you.

That was where we first glimpsed the dark tentacles holding her. With tears in my eyes, I grasped her and embraced her, gently, so grateful that we were there, and I could finally touch her. I pushed back and took her face gently between my hands and looked into her eyes. She instantly closed them and put her head down, so I released her immediately and pulled her back into my arms, hugging her ever so tightly. We stood like that for minutes, swaying slightly side to side. I just wanted to feel her, hold her, and love her.

Then I lifted my head to look at each of these people, two men and one woman, these strangers, all embracing Jesse. We swapped and it was Jesse's turn to embrace his sister while I hugged those most beautiful people. The girl was crying and didn't let me go for a long while. I joined in with tears of relief and sadness. It was not hard to determine which face belonged to Houssain. We embraced the longest, then I looked at him and thanked him.

It wasn't until later that I realised that they had literally saved our daughter's life.

Then I was able to look at our girl, really look at her.

She looked like she had not slept, showered, or taken care of herself in days. She was wearing a dress that was inside out. On top of that was a skirt, around her neck and half of her head was what looked like a large scarf. Her hair poked out and what I could see was a tangled mess. She neither knew nor cared. Her eyes were vacant.

The decline in her health in twenty-four hours was obvious to us when she talked. No, she didn't talk, she mumbled, so quietly.

We could not hear her and couldn't understand what she said. I looked at Houssain and he shrugged, his face turned sad.

She knew who we were and seemed … I would like to say she was happy to see us, but there was a nothingness about her … a wariness that I didn't understand.

She would not let go of my hand, or maybe I didn't want to let go of hers.

She kept looking at my hands and mumbled again.

I asked her, "Are you okay?"

I needed to turn my ear to her mouth and lean in close to hear what she was saying, I had to listen carefully.

"They have stolen your jewellery!" she mumbled.

"No, no," I replied. "I left my jewellery at home." I wondered who *they* were?

She muttered something again. I could make out that she thought that bad people were going to steal my jewellery, blow up our plane and kill us – if we even made it into the country. My heart skipped a beat. In no way did I imagine that this would be what we were walking into.

"Alice, nothing bad has happened, we are safe."

We were then jostled by people walking past us, and the connection between us was broken. I looked up to Jesse and noticed the others were all watching us and waiting patiently. Introductions were briefly made on the go as we started moving towards the exit.

When we reached the car park, I went with Baseem to pay the parking fee. He would not accept my money, but I was insistent and felt a small sense of victory as I handed some money to the man at the ticket booth and walked back to the car where the three friends sat in the front. Bassem was driving, Houssain was in the passenger seat and between them Kholod was wedged half on the hand brake and half on Houssain's lap.

No words were spoken as Jesse and I immediately put Alice in the middle seat in the back between us. We then had a wild ride to the hotel, weaving in and out of traffic, windows open to pull in a breeze, all the while having some inane chat about our plane trip, Istanbul and the Turkish people on the drive to our hotel. Alice didn't join in the conversation, and whether she heard anything, I do not know.

Jesse

When you spend so much time convincing yourself that you are right, is there not the possibility that you may be wrong?

Landing in Istanbul was in some ways a relief, we were now able to come out of the complete uncertainty of the blackout that air travel causes, but it did feel like we were out of the pot and into the fire.

Almost immediately it was clear this wasn't going to be the

smooth sailing we had hoped for on the flight over. When we spotted Alice and her three friends, she saw us and immediately retreated. Not necessarily in a panicked state, but a sort of turn and burn like when you see someone you know but that you don't want to see in public. Someone from the group, probably Houssain, turned with her and guided her into the arms of Mum, and from there we walked to the car.

I was trying to notice Alice's general appearance at this stage, the first part of the mental state examination. Her clothing was colourful, though nothing matched and there was the odd food stain. Her hair had that 'just out of bed' look as if she had woken up from a big night out and hadn't looked in the mirror, and it was covered with some sort of material. All these things could be considered normal for someone past their third month of continuous travel: messy, semi-dirty clothes and a big night out, normal, right? Turing away from your mum and brother who you hadn't seen in quite some time though … less normal.

The car trip into the city was cramped, it was a small sedan with not much room for six fully grown people. It wasn't a mistake, but it had taken that many of them to be able to convince Alice that going to the airport was a good idea, such was the delusional and paranoid state of mind Alice was in. Despite this crowding, the car was relatively silent on the way in, with Mum and Alice mainly just quietly holding hands. As we got closer to our destination, which was thankfully only a few hundred metres from where Houssain and the rest of the friends had been staying, the conversation became a bit easier and we were told what some of the landmarks were along the way, or where the group liked to hang out in parks or by the Bosporus. Alice was still virtually silent, trapped in her head and trapped in 'the Bull'.

CHAPTER 7

Flashback: Suma Beach

A few weeks earlier

Alice

Ashraf and his group of friends were going to Suma Beach to see Nicolás Jaar, an electronic artist, and asked me if I wanted to join them. My Aussie friend Abbey was volunteering at the hostel so she couldn't go but I was as free as a bird. So, with only minor persuasion from Houssain, we set off out of Istanbul on a drive that would take just over an hour depending on the traffic. We were in a five-seat car, with six of us squashed inside, excited and hyped for the festival.

At the festival, Houssain and Ashraf helped an American girl who had taken a bit too much ecstasy, but otherwise that night was fun. We all had a good boogie and headed back to our campsite after Jaar's set.

The day after the festival we woke up on the boiling hot sand. It was perfect weather for a morning swim. I was the first in. After that Ashraf started playing his guitar, and we spent the day relaxing, listening to music, singing and enjoying the water. Sadly, I ended up getting so sunburnt my face swelled up.

The state of the beach was quite horrendous, with rubbish littered on every part of it. I remember the day before a friend had offered me some pills and I had taken them, looking back now I wonder if it was more Captogon but I cannot recall even asking what they were. I was worried that once that they hit me, I would feel this surge of energy and need to clean the beach up, an impossible task alone!

Almost a month later, it was time for another trip to Suma Beach for a festival and this time Abbey could come. It was an hour-long trip on a ferry to Burgazada Island where we camped on the beach and visited Bassem's place on the Asian side of Istanbul. At this point I was starting to feel really scattered in my thoughts. We had plans to go back to Suma to see a meteor shower and I nearly didn't go because my brain was feeling mixed up and I felt somewhat depressed. I put it down to a combination of socialising too much and a lack of sleep.

Meanwhile, Abbey, Manar, Edwin and I returned to Avni's studio in Istanbul where Manar was able to translate from Turkish to English for us. We learnt a little about Avni's life and found out about a childhood romance that broke his heart. There was only one painting from that time in his life and it was dark and full of curves, a memento of love and loss. Avni's nephew brought us in tea and biscuits. Avni asked Abbey and me to stay at his apartment down the road if we would clean it and cook for him. I thought this was a lovely offer. We went to look at his apartment and, though it was small, I ended up moving out of the hostel to stay with the Syrians, primarily to stay with Houssain.

The main delusions that I remember came trickling in at different times. I would always wake up earlier than Houssain. During this time, I would edit the books I brought away with me, *The Dhammapada*, collected sayings of the Buddha, and *The Seven Spiritual Laws of Success* by Deepak Chopra. I was amazed I hadn't thought of erasing words as a way of reading.

These morning reflections gave me time to think of what had gone on the previous day. Perhaps too much. I wonder if it got my brain working too quickly.

Some people who have been through psychosis find it hard to get a grip on reality afterwards. They might reject what they once would have described as synchronicity (meaningful coincidences). In reality, the flavour of your life changes after you have psychosis, as you have perceived so much that wasn't tangibly there. The knowledge may be stuffed inside you and might feel quite bitter. All your once hidden fears, anxieties and insecurities have been uprooted from when they started manifesting in real time in the form of aural and visual hallucinations, for example.

Once, I spent an excessive amount of time telling my life story to the voices in my head, to the underground group around Istanbul that was tuned in to the frequency of my thoughts. One main gentleman would listen and pass on what I was saying 'down the line' so that my message would blossom and blow like the seeds of an infinitely growing flower.

Another time, voices in my head yelled at me to show him by dancing. I did not know how. I still feel a sort of disconnect remembering how saddened and confused I was by being unable to take the advice from the voices screaming in my head, it seemed entirely disrespectful to ignore them.

I joked around with Houssain about being a hippy, saying things like, "Spirit likes pineapples because of their prickly exterior and naturally sweet centre." It felt strangely relaxing to refer to myself as Spirit. The next day I found myself wondering about what my spirit name would be. Sahara came to me. It was like my middle name, Sarah. In fact, it was my mum's name jumbled up just with an extra 'a'. I wondered about the definition of each syllable in the word (Sa, Ha and Ra). Ha is filled with meaning in Sanskrit, and I took a fancy to drawing Ha on my body – in Sanskrit it kind of looks like 'cAT' without the 'A'.

This was when things slowed down a lot before they sped up real fast.

***

2 August 2015

One afternoon we decided to leave and go to the island for the second time to camp the night. In my bag I bought cumin, half an onion and some biscuits. I had never enjoyed cumin, but for some reason I had stumbled upon it in the pantry and had become fascinated by it. I would have it with everything. I had also just recently tried to take a bite out of an onion, and I would, in a couple of days, eat a raw egg whole and feel like I had just consumed a universe.

This beach where we camped didn't have the conservative feeling of the rest of Istanbul, it seemed quite free and alternative. When I arrived on the beach, I had this light feeling like people could sense my intense, awakened energy because they had already been enlightened so they knew what the feeling was like to meet another with this same awakening.

I felt like they asked, "When did she wake up?" like I was an embryo before that. A girl with dreadlocks responded, 'I could feel her energy when she walked onto the beach.' That voice and that memory to this day still feels genuine.

The stones on the beach lightly hurt my feet but it was worth it when I had the opportunity to swim. I love swimming and was keen to get in the water and I went for a two-hour swim where I experienced so many sensations. It was the first time in the sea since having this 'awakening' and I would sometimes feel like I was swimming like a seal, and then at times like a dolphin. Diving up and down in the cool water. Twirling and swirling below sea level. At the midway point of the swim, I came onto land through the soggy mesh of seaweed that covered the stones. When I looked up there was a cliff face so I climbed up it and sat on the ledge in the middle, remembering my Australian friend Micca, who would love to climb.

I swam back, slowly cruising with the current. When I was

almost to shore, a giant flock of birds, which I discovered later is called a murmuration, was cruising around in the sky. For over ten minutes this went on, and it felt totally mystical. I took it as a symbol for migration, as just before the birds split up, they made the shape of Australia. I should have called out, "Hey, doesn't that look like Australia?" but I didn't because I was so entranced by the movie-like scene unfolding before my eyes. I wondered if it meant there is going to be a mass migration to Australia?

When I eventually got back to the others, I told them what an amazing time I had, but they did not seem that impressed or interested. They weren't even inspired by what they had just seen. I felt like the vibes in the group were negative. I spoke to Amroo, who had arrived when I had been in the water. He said he had gone and got his car fixed (it stalled a few times when we were on the way to the festival) and that there was a problem with the ignition that took all day to find. I took this as a metaphor for how he was disconnected from the feminine divine. He had come onto me a couple of weeks earlier, despite knowing Houssain and I were dating. Since that night, his car had been experiencing starter problems.

Anyway, after my swim, Houssain wouldn't talk to me for some reason and Batool suggested going for a walk, so we went up the road and started picking some figs. The trees must have been on someone's property as an old lady ran towards us yelling and waving her arms, we took that as a sign to run away too. On our walk, Batool told me that I had apparently been swimming for a very long time, which is why the vibes of the group were quite sombre when I had returned. In their eyes, I had been missing. And no one could swim but me, so they were all freaking out about my swimming alone and that worry and concern grew the longer I was away from them. They were starting to worry that I had drowned.

Batool decided she was leaving and not staying the night. I decided to go too. We had dinner in the village on the island before boarding the boat. I remember thinking I'd owe her one, because she had paid for me as I had no cash left. Here we were talking, and she said it was like there was a wind in this place that changed the atmosphere, and you simply could not be out when the 'air of Istanbul' changed. Only the women felt it.

Before I left Istanbul, I gave Batool a gift to return the favour. It was a medallion that said 'immigration' in Arabic. I hope the token brings her all the luck in the world.

The next day I woke up early and put on a movie. I was looking forward to the guys getting home from the island. They came home later than I expected, and in a less calm mood than I would have anticipated. They had been in a fight with locals on the island who ran a bar. The beach was now roped off because of the conflict. Houssain came back with a cut on his arm just where I had drawn something on him the day before. It felt like things were aligning. Batool and I had left the night before because of our women's intuition that something was not right. A part of me didn't believe the brawl was real. In fact, I felt like it was a lie to intimidate me.

Unfortunately, hearing about the brawl did not diminish my elevated mood and I was unable to help Houssain clean the house, instead feeling like I needed to have my own time. Kholod came over and helped clean also, but I just could not do it, instead choosing to embrace my elevated mood and remain detached from people with a lower mood. I could not understand why this was.

CHAPTER 8

Downtown Istanbul

Monday 31 August 2015

Sarah

It was around 2 pm when we arrived at our hotel and the afternoon was hot and sticky. The hotel was squeezed tightly between apartment blocks that were three stories high. We retrieved my suitcase from the car and Jesse arranged to meet Houssain in thirty minutes to ask more about what has gone on with Alice. The plan was that later we would all go over to pick up Alice's belongings at the apartment. We gave a heartfelt thanks to Bassem for interrupting his day to collect us from the airport. He could see how grateful we were, but I suspect he did it more to help out his friends who were at a loss of what to do about Alice and how to get her to the airport safely and without incident.

I checked in to our hotel as quickly and efficiently as possible while Jesse stayed outside with a listless Alice. To get to our room on the second floor we needed to squeeze the three of us and our luggage into the tiniest of lifts that was meant to be for two people. The hotel apartment consisted of three rooms. The entrance door opened to a little kitchenette, a fridge, a microwave, and a table with four chairs that sat on a small Turkish rug. To one side there was a tiny room with a fold up bed that was for Jesse to sleep on and also there was a television on the wall. An old bathroom divided the rooms. The last room was for Alice and me. It was a sun-filled room with a large window. In it was a king size bed, a wardrobe and a door that led out to a set of rickety stairs down to the courtyard that we could see from our window.

Jesse dragged my luggage to the bedroom and I put the kettle on for a cuppa. Then we all flopped on the bed exhausted and asked Alice how she was. She didn't know the answer to this, the simplest of questions. I suspect we had arrived with barely a moment to spare.

She whispered that she didn't like it if I looked into her eyes, so I didn't. I was not sure why this scared her so much, perhaps she thought I could see into her soul.

Only a couple of hours had gone by since arriving, but we were gleaning bits and pieces of information to fill in the puzzle of what was going on in her mind.

If it was scary for us, it must have been truly terrifying for her.

Our girl did not like all the noises going on around her, and the voices and the whirling goings on in her brain, so we gave her Jess's headphones with calming music playing from his iPod. Jesse told her that to skip a song she just had to tap a button on the lead twice. It was a stroke of genius, and this device and the music quickly became the lifeline that Alice needed. Months later, when we were home, she told us that when the voices in her head were crowding in on her, she would tap the lead and it would skip the song and help her brain lose some of the voices. It seemed to reset her mind for a short moment, if she was lucky a minute or two.

While I tried to get our girl to sleep or at least rest, Jesse left to find Houssain's apartment to get a full account from them of what had been happening with Alice.

Alice

I could barely believe it when I saw Mum and Jesse appear at the airport. I noticed Mum didn't have jewellery on and I wondered if she had to give them to the terrorists to be here with me. I believed that she had to have sex with many famous band members to get to Istanbul. The reason was to keep me safe. I also knew that Jesse and Mum had to live multiple past lives in discomfort to be here for me now. This placed an immense burden on me. They both looked exhausted. That day I believed I had to live for all human spirits to survive an alien invasion. I would be plagued with dreams from the alien fugitives.

CHAPTER 9

Flashback: the kitten

A few weeks before

Alice

I'd been keeping an eye on the street cat situation, watching from the balcony and the window in the kitchen. One of them looked like my cat Rumi. I was taking a shower one morning and, for whatever reason, I started singing *The Lion King*'s intro song. I hadn't sung that or seen the movie in years, so I didn't know where it came from. When I got out of the shower, I went into the kitchen to make a cup of tea. I noticed there was a street cat with her kitten at the window. I opened it and the mother left. I spent three days with this kitten.

Just to encapsulate a little of my energy and enthusiasm, here is what I messaged my mum:

I got a kitten!! It's perfect, it's soooo sooo chill. It just gets me! I knew when she was on the windowsill that this is a good one. It took a while to warm up to me. But I knew it was worth it and it was a completely natural process. Nature's gift!!

Funny how I had just had a shower and sang the song from *The Lion King*! How's that for in sync with nature?

I texted Raha (a friend in Sydney) about it and she said she had just literally thought how she wanted a kitten. I recalled that the day before I was walking home from the grocery and saw a cat inside an apartment and I thought, *Wow, a cat inside, not fair I want one.*

The kitten was a street cat and very hesitant to let me near but the minute I put a ribbon around its neck it came over to sit on my lap! Amazing. I called the kitten Saha.

It came to be that the more time I spent with the kitten, the more I realised how many things there are to think about and discuss. Especially after being around people speaking another language so often around me. One of my anxieties back at the beginning of the trip was that I sometimes didn't know what to say in group situations, I felt more of an observer than a participant. Now it seemed so clear to me that the issue began deep within, when I hadn't taken enough time to check in with thoughts and feelings, instead turning to marijuana to even out the interesting thoughts and numb the more painful thoughts effortlessly. And now here I was, with a super-mellow friendly gift from nature. Thinking how lovely it was to have a kitten to pat and look after. I noticed on the first evening with the kitten that she had a piece of glass, or a crystal, stuck inside her foot. I was able to get it out with tweezers, then I poured some vodka on it to cleanse it. It seemed to sting her for a few seconds but then she licked it up and it looked a lot cleaner.

Later that night we were sitting in Ashraf's room, a group of about seven of us, and I thought I'd like to jot down what happened this morning with the kitten. I wrote a little bit, then I put down my journal, thinking, *It can wait till tomorrow, I just want to be here with the group now*. About fifteen minutes later I picked up my journal to see what I had written, and all I wrote was 'Today I woke up'. I found this hilarious and laughed till I cried. No one else seemed to find it as funny as I did. I took it as a very deep appreciation of the nature of the self. It was something I'd never been able to laugh at before. Thinking I wanted to write about an event, and only writing, 'I woke up'. Hilarious! That night the group went out clubbing and I stayed home to be with the kitten and have time to think. I remembered wanting to go out but not wanting to do the walk alone.

The next night, Manar brought some friends over from the hostel. We all had a good chat and passed around the kitten. At some point during the night, though, the kitten vanished and that was goodbye. I remember that night I tried to give the Deepak Chopra book away to a girl and her sister, but the older sister said she had read it and had a copy at home. I thought I could tell that she had read it ...

***

Thursday 27 August 2015

At first it was only the voices of two people I had met in Bulgaria. They seemed like very spiritually liberated people so it makes sense that the delusions would take hold through them. I remember Houssain asking me who I was talking to and I said their names. He replied, "It sounds like you're talking to imaginary friends." I was defensive as I didn't think it was imaginary.

Later, I believed that I was being monitored by the couple that had managed the hostel in Bulgaria and that they were overseeing my expression or degree of spirituality via implanting the kitten with a crystal in its foot. This crystal was returned to them when the cat vanished so that they could gauge my care of it using some new form of technology that could read levels of love in nature and nurture. It was about this time that I noticed a strange wire sitting on the table where a piece of smoky quartz was sitting. I somehow had the feeling that I was not only monitored by the Bulgarian couple, but I was also being looked at by the French who were possibly paying Bassem to be an informer …

I had bought the smoky quartz from a crystal shop in the Grand Bazaar where I would spend up to an hour and a half at a time, observing the people coming and going, observing the employees with their little knowledge of the stock they were selling. I got lost in the crystal store and came to love this smoky quartz piece so much that I returned to get it days after first seeing it. It was destined to be smashed, turns out.

A couple of days after the self-proclaimed naming (Sahara) and the reception of the kitten, I needed to listen to Koori Radio, so I streamed it online. This made me feel super relaxed, so laid back that I began to draw all over my face. I sent an image and a video to Mum, in which I was on such a natural high, I said, "Can I be Australia's next top model yet?" and mocked how I auditioned for it in previous years. I found this hilarious. I felt like I had this lightness of being about me, and that I was just starting to see myself as I truly am. I was able to just be high on life ...

CHAPTER 10

Impressions of Alice

Monday 31 August 2015

Sarah

While Jesse was out, I barricaded the doors of the hotel room. I put my suitcase and Alice's backpack against one of the doors that led down to the communal garden outside our room. The chairs from the kitchen went in front of the hotel room door and, as a last line of defence, the little lock chain on the door was attached. I did this hoping that if she tried to leave, one of us would hear her and be able to stop her.

I took time to think how luck, strangely, was on our side. How blessed we were that she had had friends looking after her that cared enough to contact a family all the way across the world, Syrian friends that were refugees themselves. Fate, providence, or just good fortune that Alice found a wonderful man like Houssain. How amazing it was that he was there to help Alice and protect her when she needed it.

Houssain had been through unimaginable physical and mental trauma in Syria. The sorrow of leaving his homeland, separated from his family and friends. Yet there he was staying with her and saving our girl.

I thought how fortunate she was that Jesse and I were able to make it there to get her.

When we were in the bedroom, she whispered that she had caused much upheaval for us. That it would be better if she was not there at all. I didn't want to ask her what she meant by that. I was too scared to hear whatever might be the answer. My heart broke yet again, and I held her ever so closely. So tightly. I looked at her and said, "I promise you; I will never let you go."

I am not sure if she understood or could hear me through the voices in her head, but regardless, she hugged me back.

The tentacles were starting to wrap tightly around her. I wanted to rip them off, but I didn't know how.

I settled Alice into bed and suggested she had a little 'nanna nap'. Softly, I told her I was not going anywhere. After closing the connecting sliding door, I put the kettle on and sat at the table with my head in my hands and had a little cry. I was exhausted but so relieved to be there and have Alice in a safe place.

I went and sat on Jesse's bed, it was one of those beds that is made from a two-seater lounge, one end of which has pull out legs but when I sat on it, it collapsed, and I crashed to the ground with a thud! When Jesse returned, we tried to fix it but couldn't seem to manage to correct the problem. It was quite amusing and that ended up being how Jesse slept that night, head up and feet virtually on the ground as we couldn't work out how to put it up properly. For some reason, we didn't think to ask the front desk for help!

After I picked myself up from the floor, I got up to have a sneak peek at Alice. I quietly opened the sliding door dividing the kitchen and entrance to our bedroom. I had a heart attack because Alice was standing right at the door, literally a centimetre from it. Eyes closed, arms raised above her head with her elbows out and hands clasped together in some sort of yoga or prayer pose. I think I must have jumped a foot in the air and my heart raced. I definitely swore and a nervous giggle escaped from me. I asked her if she was okay. She nodded with vacant, tired eyes and I guided her back to bed, lay her down and stroked her hair. I had no idea what else to do.

Jesse

We sorted out the bed situation in the hotel room – Mum to share the king with Alice, and myself on the pull-out in the other room. All this decision-making provided further insight into Alice's mental state. I asked her a few questions while we were sorting out the hotel room. She seemed worried but told me she was calm and happy that we were there but seemed confused as to why. She told me she felt safe but I was not convinced. She also kept calling Istanbul 'the Bull'. I thought this must have been a common nickname for the place, but later would find out this was essentially her pet name for the prison she had found herself in, in her own mind, but in the city of Istanbul, 'the Bull'.

Once Mum and Alice were settled, I went to speak with Alice's friends and housemates to hear exactly what had been going on from their point of view over the last few weeks in Istanbul. Houssain walked with me from the hotel to the apartment to see the same group of people who were with us in the car. We started with some small talk initially before I gave my spiel that we were going to get Alice home and that I needed to have as much information that they could tell me as possible. I wanted to better understand her deterioration in mental health to that point.

I heard the story of how they all met, what they did in the beginning together and when they thought Alice had begun to change. All of them in some way or another had attributed the Captagon to either all or part of her decline. They were angry with their so-called friend that had given the pill to her. In fact, they had two other close friends who had similar stories of mental breakdown or psychosis. They were also acutely aware of Captogon use and abuse in the war that had displaced them from their homes. Though that is another story in itself. Trauma, vulnerability and neurotoxic drugs.

These people had seen it all, had seen too much. I felt like they had all also lost so much. Their kindness and bravery in summoning our family showed that they were not willing to lose any more. I heard consistently about Alice's gradual decline, from happy-go-lucky to paranoid and deluded. From sweet and cuddly to violent and aggressive. The list could go on and on but the message was staying the same, regardless of the cause, Alice was unwell and in the grips of a real-life, full-blown psychosis. The rose-tinted glasses were smashed off my face. Red flags abounded and they all signalled one thing: get her home.

With hugs and thanks for all they had done for my sister, I left and headed back to the hotel. I needed to speak to Mum later that night when Alice was asleep.

After a quick nap, Alice, Mum and I ventured back down the road to where Alice had been staying. We helped Alice collect her belongings from the last month. Pack her life up, it seemed as well. The apartment was in the lower ground floor of a typical multilevel apartment building in Istanbul that were tall and thin, much like those of northern Europe. There were five Syrian refugees and Alice staying in the apartment, the common room having a spare bed as well. It looked like any regular share house you would find in any city of the world containing five mid-to-late-twenties people.

We had a quick tour of the place and sat down with Alice, Houssain and two of the other housemates. At that stage it was all a pretty normal interaction. There was tea and coffee, some Australian chocolate biscuits, Tim Tams. We showed them how to drink coffee through the biscuit. This caused a bit of spilled coffee too, but worth it to hear the laughter that abounded. When we tried to get them to eat Vegemite, they had clearly heard of it or maybe even tasted it and were not to be persuaded to try it this time.

Alice was mainly silent.

We were wrapping up our afternoon and planning to go back to the hotel to take stock when Alice showed her first glimpse of the proper erratic activity that had caused her friends to contact us in the first place. She suddenly stood up and went to Houssain's room and began tearing it apart rather unceremoniously to find something. Something that she could not explain beyond that she needed to find it. After some carnage from the search, a small piece of cardboard was found that had some of Alice's scribbles on it, some indecipherable scribble and some peculiar, nonsensical sentences that could not have been so important to require flipping your friend's bedroom to find. We were eventually able to leave with evidence rapidly mounting to bring her back home.

On the walk back to the hotel, Mum had dropped Alice's hand to fix a bag she was carrying and Alice, seeing an opportunity, tried to run away. I dropped her backpack and was able to grab her before she had got to far down the street. My adrenaline was pumping, I grasped her and pulled her into an embrace, and said, "Everything's okay. We are here. Look, there's Mum."

Mum of course hugged her and said, "You gave us a big fright, Al. Don't run away from us. We are here to help you."

Mum and I looked at each other and I mouthed, *Bloody hell!*

When we asked her why she had done that, she couldn't explain her actions. Her disorganised thoughts were plain to see.

Sarah

On returning from Houssain's, I got some fresh clothes out of Alice's bag and set her up in the shower with soap, shampoo and conditioner. I asked if she was ok to wash her hair and she looked at me expressionlessly. "I can wash it for you, you get started." I squirted some liquid soap onto her hands and told her to wash her body and, like a robot, she did. A simple shower took longer than expected.

By the time she had finished, the three of us were extremely hungry and tired. The decision was made to go find a place for dinner. Alice wanted to take us somewhere, but ten minutes after we left the hotel, we were hopelessly lost.

Five short days ago, she was very familiar with these streets. But that day she was like a computer wiped clean of all information, a blank walking, talking (or rather mumbling) human.

We finally came across a group of six very crowded restaurants, jampacked with a mixture of what looked like tourists and locals. We chose the only restaurant with a table vacant outside. That was our first experience with Alice and crowds in her new state.

We ordered food and drinks immediately. The waiter brought a carafe of water and three glasses. Turkish coffee was ordered for Jess and we leaned back in our chairs, at least Jesse and I did, to try and relax and enjoy the atmosphere. Alice could usually be considered a coffee snob, and Jess was excited to try authentic Turkish coffee and so he asked Alice what she thought of it. She said, in her quiet little voice, that she didn't know, and that she hadn't tried it. That was surprising and definitely not true. Alice said it with such conviction, as in her mind that was the reality, there was no coffee in the Bull.

A restful dinner turned out to be impossible, as within minutes of ordering, Alice became fidgety and anxious. Her eyes started darting from side to side, her left leg jiggled, and she suddenly stood up and turned to leave, forgetting that we were with her or that we even existed. I stood and grabbed her arm, flinging my other arm over her shoulders.

"Where are you going, Belle?" I reverted to a sweet name I used to call Alice when she was a child.

"I do not like it, I am going." Alice was not looking at us when she was speaking.

"How about you stay? The food is just about here, and we will eat it, then walk back home," Jess said this so matter-of-factly and in such a firm, no-nonsense voice that Alice did as she was directed.

Good fortune was on our side as, no sooner had he said this, the food and coffee arrived and we ate as fast as we could. Me with my hand on Alice's thigh and watching her like a hawk and Jesse trying to savour and enjoy his first authentic Turkish coffee, with one eye on Alice and the other so wanting to soak up the atmosphere.

It was a bad move to go out for dinner, but we did and we needed to make a positive of it. We finished dinner in record time. Sadly, I cannot even recall what we ate or what it tasted like. I paid the bill while Jess looked longingly at the Turkish coffee being drunk leisurely at the next table. Then we left.

Jesse asked Alice if she thought she could find her way back to Houssain's, then we would know how to get back to the hotel from there.

"Sure, follow me." She said that ever so quietly, in a monotone voice. No inflection. No pitch. No … nothing.

We walked around for about twenty minutes until Jesse and I looked at each other and nodded our heads in recognition that we were heading in circles. We realised that Al had no idea where she was or where she was going.

Fortunately, Jesse got us in the right direction and finally home, exhausted but safe.

Earlier that day, when we were walking to Houssain's, then to dinner and later eating out, I learnt that when Alice started squeezing my hand, she was nervous, confused or totally unsure of herself.

Most of the time we held hands, or my arm was around her shoulders, reassuring her or perhaps myself that she was grounded and safe. Whenever she squeezed my hand, I squeezed her hand back to reassure her. If I am honest, I needed it too.

The jiggling of her thighs I had not yet worked out but perhaps it was the psychosis, anxiety or both.

I got Alice's teeth brushed, pyjamas on and put her into bed. With the doors locked, bags and chairs were then put back against the doors, making her potential exit noisy and time-consuming, if she was to make it that far.

We feel like we needed eyes in the back of our heads. We were seriously under siege from the delusions and voices that were playing havoc with Alice's brain. When I was getting Alice into bed, she told me the voices in her head overwhelmed her. I tried hard to think of something positive to say, but my mind went blank. I pulled her into my arms and hugged her tight. At that moment, show don't tell seemed to be the way to go.

All the while my heart was breaking into a million pieces watching her mind fall apart right before my eyes.

Alice

Going out to dinner with Mum and Jesse was not a pleasant experience for me. Fortunately, the music playing in my head, through Jesse's headphones, was better than listening to the voices. They did not cease altogether, though, but it was at least a respite.

The people on the street freaked me out on our way to dinner and I became quite anxious. My delusions were confused, and I was struggling to keep a grip on reality, although I clearly had no reality to grasp onto. The one constant was Mum holding my hand or my arm. When we sat down at the table, I was horrified because I saw the waiter put an enormous plate of poo on the table with the water, I wanted to get away from there but Mum would not let me go. They sat there eating their food oblivious to what was on the table, while I sat and watched them in stunned silence.

Sarah

When Alice was in bed, Shane, Jesse and I had a three-way conversation on when to come home. Sadly, it was blatantly obvious after returning from Houssain's and then dinner that Alice's behaviour and the uncertainty with the voices in her head meant that we would be flying home sooner rather than later.

I started laughing and crying telling them about finding Alice's face and body practically imprinted on the door when I had gone to check on her earlier. Jesse hugged me but I told him that it was also pretty funny and started laughing again, grateful to be able to giggle at my own expense about how much it freaked me out finding her like that. We all laughed at the inanity of it all. It lightened the mood and released a bit of our own nervous tension.

Then I looked back at my messages and re-read one from Houssain that had gone unnoticed. I showed Jesse with raised eyebrows and messaged Houssain immediately.

I'm so sorry I missed your text about why you were picking us up at the airport. How was Alice dangerous?

Dangerous, like she started being violent.

Oh my God! What did she do?

She ran away and tried several times to get in a car with strangers. She hit me when I tried to prevent her from getting in the random cars. But at some point, she comes back to reality and say things meaning that she realised that she is having a weird experience and she is fighting it.

Are you okay? Thank God you were able to stop her but I'm so shocked to hear that she tried to hurt you!

Sarah, she was not in her right mind, but she is trying to fight it.

My God, we owed this man Alice's life.
More pieces of this horrible puzzle were coming together.
My heart was heavy, this was not going to be a quick fix for our darling girl.

Decision made, Jesse got on his computer, and we started booking our return trip home. Our dinner excursion was the catalyst that we needed to make the correct and only decision. It was essential to get her home to medical treatment.

A flight out of Istanbul's Atatürk Airport was found through Singapore Airlines, leaving on Wednesday at around lunchtime. There would be nearly eleven hours flight time to Singapore then a stopover at the airport before a further seven-hour flight home to Sydney. Around twenty hours, and the unknown of how Alice would cope with being in an enclosed space in the air.

Later that night, when I went to bed, Alice was awake and looked terrified. I asked her if she could tell me what was going on? She thought the *doof, doof* noises of the music at the nightclub several streets away were bombs going off. She wanted to know why I wasn't concerned and got quite agitated that I was ignoring the situation. I tried to tell her that that was not happening, that we were safe and reminded her that we were in the hotel and that we would protect her. There were *NO* bombs, it was a nightclub and the thumping was the beat of the music. I have no doubt that she didn't believe me, but reassurance and honesty seemed to be the best option for me to take with Alice.

Finally, she fell into a restless sleep. I was exhausted but on high alert to any sound or movement. I was worried that if I fell asleep too deeply, she would leave. When she made little groaning noises while she slept, I assumed she was distressed. I rubbed her back, or arm or held her hand and told her everything was okay and my mantra became, "You are strong and confident, you are going to be ok.' I suspected I was saying those words for myself too, as it made me feel a little better.

***

31 August and 1 September 2015, overnight

Alice

I had talked to Mum before I went to sleep but she really did not understand me. During the night I would wake up to the sounds of bombing and I would feel it was my calling to leave the hotel and do a Cersei (a character from *Game of Thrones* who walked naked through the streets to atone). I felt like we were all stuck in the Tibetan book of the dead's Bardo (that is said to be a state of limbo after death before afterlife, dense in illusion), and that I was at the end of the helpline for people who had committed suicide. I had to survive so that their spirits would not be consumed by parasitic aliens who had arrived on earth on ships.

I couldn't do a Cersei though, Mum wasn't letting me go anywhere by myself unless it was to the bathroom.

The voices were hard to ignore. What did it mean to be the end of a help line for those who had committed suicide? It meant that I was full. I believed the afterlife was full, too. This energy, this fullness, was indicative of my mentality being overloaded with information, stimuli and thoughts.

CHAPTER 11

Flashback: Trouble in Istanbul

Monday 10 August 2015

Alice

One night Mehmed and a friend of his came over. I had just had the idea that everything needs an equal and opposite reaction, and that there is a transaction fee to those before us who have created various technological devices. For example, to open the fridge one might need to dance around the kitchen or something. Mehmed and his friend didn't understand.

I also had the belief that you could figure out answers by staring at your left eye in the mirror. I'm not sure what I asked myself but perhaps this delusion helped me uncover another delusion, that by thinking of two people and a landmark or building, you could contact higher dimensional beings. I would often think of a friend called Tia, who had just been to Egypt to visit some family members, and Lozza or Ella, and pair them with the Great Pyramid or Uluru. Doing this sometimes felt like a mental stretch, like a way to foster strength and resilience.

We were on the way to Batool's house, and we stopped at the shops to buy some food. I remember feeling anxious and on edge when this was happening. The streets freaked me out. Just being outside induced fear in me.

At first, I think this was because I felt how unhappy Houssain was in Istanbul, but as we walked around, I noticed how invasive the signs on the streets were and how intense the people were, not smiling but not quite resting bitch-face. I did not think it was simply because I was generally more anxious.

The lady at the counter barely said anything to us and she dropped 25 cents of our change on the floor. This stressed me out because the twenty-fifth is my birthday. We stepped into another store, and the guy at the counter there also dropped 25 cents of our change. This made me believe that there was a bigger picture going on in the city here, and it made me wonder if it was supernatural forces at hand that had brainwashed the people of Istanbul. This would eventually contribute to my feeling of being stuck in limbo, in the Bardo of the Bull. I also had a belief that nothing really happens unless it happens twice. Perhaps this stems from a loosely based yin yang delusion or a belief in duality.

I also had mind-reading thoughts. At first it felt like I was transferring thoughts to people, and they could relay thoughts to other people. It was like I was telling my story. At Batool's house I was sitting on the toilet and there was no toilet paper. I stayed there for a long time, believing I was telling my story to people in close proximity. It wasn't the voice of people from the hostel in Bulgaria anymore, it was a network of other people. I believed it was an underground movement.

I was transmitting thoughts to Batool when I was in the room with her. For example, Houssain was talking and I made a joke about him in my mind but didn't voice it, and Batool looked at me and we laughed. I believed I asked Batool if Houssain knew about this wave of thinking, and she said no. I tried to help induct him into the spiritual group that we were, by a meditation using a bag I bought from a second-hand store in Istanbul. The bag had a design shaped like Australia on it, with curvy lines decorating the coastline. I believed that this line had to be felt with the index finger, from the top to the bottom, and repeated back the way you came. Voices yelled at me to describe with body language, but I didn't know how I could do the dance I thought they wanted me to. I thought these ways of communication without words (especially telepathy) existed for ages but only now had I been able to tap into it.

How unfair!

So, at first this ability to transfer thoughts was satisfying, but then it got scarier and lonely. I have never asked Batool about this incident.

A note

It took me six months to put into words what I believed was going on with Houssain. Sure, before I felt perpetually scared and afraid, the experience of losing touch with reality was quite a 'special' experience. I felt like I was chosen, like I was God and that all the events in my life had occurred so that I could meet Houssain, and together we would be an ultimate power couple that could help change the world for the better.

***

Friday 28 August 2015

I should have realised that I was getting quite mentally mixed up. One night we were lying on the bed, I looked at Houssain and he turned into a bull or a devil-like creature in front of me, so I punched him. It was the first time I had ever punched someone. It was weird for me to be aggressive, but it was like I was so numb to the fact that something had drastically changed in me. I know now that that was a side effect of Captagon, and it only seemed to get worse from there. From that night onwards I became afraid of sleep.

It was that night that I believed Houssain was asking me to transgress reality with him. The idea was planted in my brain by Manar who earlier in the day had asked if I had heard about the Greeks who copulated and could walk on a higher dimension of reality, or something like that. Later on, I wrote about this experience in my journal:

> *Oh, my goodness, the page won't turn. I'm here in Ashraf's room wondering when I will leave. The only thing that exists is me and him. It is as though he is an alien and I am his postcard. I*

send this to myself to vent the toxins of about twelve hours spent underground living a real dreamtime. Like Greek Gods copulating in glitter. Real.

In reality, the experience was not as glorified as it felt. It was quite intimidating as I felt like I couldn't leave the room. I was frozen in the room because I was entranced by Ashraf's presence, paired with a huge curiosity of what Manar had said earlier in the day. Whatever the transgression meant, I refused because I would not leave my family who were on the other side of the world. I would not leave my family who seemed so far, unreal and distant … a fading support line.

Everything had meaning. What if how you have things positioned on your bedside table has a specific correlation to the frequency of another planet? If you impact another planet somewhere when you move something into a position, or remove it? One night I thought that it was signalling to me that my friends survived the Syrian conflict because they knew how to manipulate alternative dimensions, and that they received help from somewhere in the cosmos so they were able to leave the conflict zones.

At some point I became scared very quickly. I felt like our power combined was detected by a drone placed inside Houssain by the government when he was put in jail during the Syrian revolution for attempting to take photographs at a rally. So, it was known in my mind that the Syrian government was onto us, and we were going to be abducted. I thought people could hear what I was thinking and that Houssain was fighting a powerful battle between good and bad forces, and he wasn't sure if he could protect me from the bad forces that had intruded on his life because of his short-lived time in jail.

I became really scared one night after I asked Houssain what happened to him in Syria. When he was finished his story, I realised that I had no idea what he had said, I had zoned out completely. I was so scared of what I had missed in the conversation, and why I had zoned out. It felt like I had been put under a spell and I was being tested in our relationship and in those with my new friends, all of whom I had so much respect for.

Houssain came to realise that I was going a bit loopy. He contacted my parents. I remember that I talked with Mum and Jesse but what we discussed is not there in my brain. I felt like we were talking in code, with the subtle undertone that everything was going to be alright, that I just needed to get myself to the meeting place, I thought the plan was that there was no plan.

I was overcome with delusion and fear. By the time Mum was on her way, I fully believed that she wasn't going to make it. That she would be shot down in the airport or that the plane would be shot down before it landed by rebels. She sent a photo to me in which she looked exhausted, and I thought it was because she knew that she was flying into her own death.

***

Saturday 29 August 2015

The night before, or one of the nights before Mum arrived in Istanbul, Mohammad, Manar, and Houssain tried to get me out of the house because I hadn't been out in days. It was a full moon. I wore two dresses, one over the other, with a scarf around my neck and a hat on my head, and to top it all off I had a T-shirt over the dress. I was visually a mess, but I thought I had been having some spiritual experience.

If I wasn't so delusional, I would have recognised the symptoms of anxiety and the extreme paranoia I was feeling.

I know now that because these people were relatively new in my life, it was obvious that I didn't have as deep a connection with them as I thought. I had heard my new friends' stories of separation from their country and forced schisms with their families. I felt so sad that I had no strength to ask more about their escape from Syria and how they were now.

On the island of Burgazada, Mohammad explained his situation to me, about leaving his girlfriend, mother and two sisters behind in Syria. I felt like I couldn't ask questions because I didn't trust that I was worth asking them.

Overall, the experience has shown me how I was unable to be my own friend, blaming my anxiety on made-up perceptions of the world. I couldn't help but be captive to powerful delusions. I believed that my connection to the kittens and cats of Istanbul had opened a portal from the east and west and ultimately to Ancient Egypt. This is pertinent as it meant that everything was connected in my state of mind. I thought about how technology today is nowhere near as strong as the technology of the planet, the natural ways of the cyclical moon cycle, and the rising and falling of the sun in the sky every night. I believed that Ancient Egyptians had the most powerful mind control system ever known on this planet.

My brain was sick, and I needed help.

CHAPTER 12

Mum and Jesse in the Bull

Tuesday 1 September 2015

Sarah

Alice thankfully slept for five or six hours, not all at once, but from what Houssain had said, it was a step in the right direction. There was one heart-stopping moment during the night when she got up around 2 am. I awoke with a fright as I had heard a faint noise at the door of our room.

I nearly fell out of bed, legs tangled in the sheets trying to reach her, heart thumping, brain in overdrive. I grabbed her by the arm.

"What are you doing, Al?"

"I'm going out."

"No, you're not, it is night-time and we're sleeping now, come on, back to bed. Where do you want to go?"

She mumbled something that I couldn't decipher, I held my breath and gently guided her back to bed.

I knew she would have just walked out the door in her shortie pyjamas, bare feet and wild bed hair without a care in the world.

Lying down, we held hands and I stroked her forehead. I prayed that she would stay, but more importantly that she'd fall back asleep. Meanwhile, I was wide awake, slightly terrified to close my eyes and when I did start drifting off to sleep, I'd wake with a start and immediately look to Alice's side of the bed to make sure she was there. I did that a few more times before I finally fell into a longer, restless sleep.

Jesse

Unbeknownst to me in my slumber, Alice had apparently attempted to leave in the middle of the night. To where? It wasn't important, but something in her head had dictated that leaving the hotel was the correct thing to do. Mum had managed to calm the situation herself and I had slept blissfully through it. While they were sleeping after the ordeal, I had left the hotel and walked around the city as the sun rose at 5 am. I was up due to the travellers' curse of the dreaded jetlag.

The sunrise was an unbelievable assortment of the most vivid colours, reds, oranges and yellows, with splashes of purple that added to the brilliance. I only wished that Mum and Alice were there to see it with me.

When I made it down to the Galata Bridge, I witnessed the most massive murmuration of starlings that I have ever seen. The only way to describe it is millions of starlings moving as one through the sky, like smoke in a soft breeze. I know that Alice saw this occurrence during her time at the beach before we arrived. I cannot imagine what seeing this would be like to a person going through psychosis.

The writing was finally on the wall, we had now been convinced that the only path forward was to take Alice home for prompt medical care and assessment. The only reason we weren't leaving that day was because there were no flights.

The decision to go to the markets and out to dinner wasn't because we were still kidding ourselves that Alice was well enough to do these things. The pros outweighed the cons. We couldn't stay trapped in the rooms all day. We rationalised it that we only had one day to explore Istanbul. We thought that sitting around and doing nothing might allow Alice's mind to be more prone to unsafe liability. In the sterile light and white walls of the hotel it was only Alice and her disorganised thoughts.

Sarah

Alice had her music and headphones.

I had a backpack filled with bottled water and Jess held our crisp new tourist map from the hotel front desk in his hands.

Arm in arm, Alice, Jesse and I headed out along the narrow back roads that meandered through tiny streets. Cats were scattered outside nearly every apartment, lazing on the doorsteps and balconies or draped over window ledges. We walked down the hill until we got to the main road that crossed the Bosporus Strait, an axis of ancient and contemporary history.

The stroll down took us over an hour, and we were hungry and thirsty. Jess couldn't wait for the opportunity to taste another Turkish coffee and Alice didn't mind what we did, at least at that moment. We stopped at the bridge and leaned against a wall that came up to our hips and then we watched the water coursing past. Men of all ages were casting fishing lines out over the bridge. Sitting on baskets, chatting, and smoking with their friends. We were just a blip on their radar as we passed by.

To the left was a huge cruise ship that had docked. To the right, we saw hordes of people going about their daily lives. We joined back in the throng, and I clasped Alice's hand in mine, still concerned that she might make another run for it like the night before.

We wandered across the bridge to sit at one of the large tourist cafés that had a view of the water and ate some breakfast and discussed our plans for the morning.

There were two items on my list of things to do: see the Grand Bazaar and purchase some baklava. My needs were simple. Jesse wanted a Persian hall runner from the Bazaar for his apartment back in Melbourne. His want was a little more difficult to negotiate and he was mindful of Alice potentially not being able to last the distance. Our mission then was to walk through the spice markets, head straight to the bazaar and endeavour to find a rug for Jesse's apartment.

It all felt so simple.

Alice

In the daytime when we went for a walk, Jesse gave me Tame Impala's album, *Currents*, and Alpine's *Yuck* album to listen to.

He gave me his headphones and said that one tap on the cable was pause and two taps was next. I took this as literally pausing thoughts, and 'nexting' the stream of thoughts, as opposed to merely just pausing the song and playing the next track. This became a coping mechanism from that day, through to my time at USpace, and sometimes to this day I still have a one-tap-pause during a song.

I still had not pieced together that what I was experiencing was an illness, and it was terribly frightening to be in the Bull, in Bardo.

Sarah

Breakfast was a disaster. Alice simply could not sit there, her anxiety ran high and we assumed delusions were tumbling around her mind like clothes in a washing machine. We spent most of the time trying to rationalise with her to sit, that we were in no danger, but just there to have some coffee, something to eat and to enjoy the beautiful view of the Bosporus. None of that made any sense to Alice, but she couldn't verbalise what she wanted to tell us, other than with her agitated movements.

I wondered what we looked like to others. Did anyone notice us at all? In any case, no one observing us would have been aware of what was happening to our girl. There was no outside injury to see, no limp, no plaster covering a broken bone, no bandage on her beautiful head, nothing.

Jesse and I were like ducks, calm on the outside but paddling madly on the inside.

Time was clearly limited. Alice was on edge, I was anxious and exhausted and Jess was keen to see what the markets could yield. Jesse was our driving force and fuelled what was left of my positive energy.

So, on we went.

As we neared the markets, I realised we had completely underestimated that there would be so much, well, everything: noise, people, smells. I was immediately concerned about how Alice would cope with this 'everything'. The aromas were amazing, all the spices and different scents accosted us in the most wild and wonderful way. It was a hive of activity; think Sunday town markets but on steroids, lots of them!

I was not sure how long it took us to walk through the spice markets, but Jesse and I kept stopping to look at almost anything and everything. It was a technicolour dream come true. I was not sure if our girl was even seeing what we saw or if she had drifted away in her own mind.

We held hands, she squeezed my hand when she was not okay, and we'd stop.

Notwithstanding the mayhem of our situation, I realised the special place we were in and the deep history surrounding us. Just before we entered the old markets, I looked up, stood on my tippy-toes, and reached my arm as high as I could against the wall to feel the cold stone beneath my fingers and the palm of my hand just for a few seconds. Imagining that no one else had touched that exact spot since 1455 when parts of the Grand Bazaar were first built.

The crowd had thinned a little as we entered the bazaar. The bright sunlight from outside was suddenly blanketed by the ancient city walls. There was cold stone beneath our feet and vibrant shops beside us where tourists browsed and sellers plied their trade.

'Nearly-doc', Jesse, knew the colours of the rug that he wanted and the price that he could afford, which wasn't much. We went into a few shops, learned to negotiate, and moved on, until we found a shop that looked right. The owner could sense a sale and came in for the hard sell … with Turkish tea. He talked of a cousin who lived in Melbourne, his English was flawless and his salesmanship well-polished from years of experience.

He sat us down, brought out the tea and started the show, rolling out hall runners. The first one he showed was absolutely beautiful, the colours were amazing, with greens, pinks and that beautiful azure blue but at $10,000 it was sadly a no from us. I could not help but look at Jesse and we laughed out loud, which brought a wry smile and a little shrug from the seller.

Finally, Jess saw the one and nodded to the seller, the negotiations started at $3000, laughably he only had $600 to spend.

The bartering happened, the boss dropped his price to $1500 and – God bless her – at the crucial part of negotiations Alice got up to walk out. I grabbed her hand and stood up beside her.

I whispered quietly into Alice's ear, trying to soothe her from what was whirling around in her brain.

The boss was watching us, then Jesse, then back to us. No doubt he thought that a sale and all his hard work was about to walk out the door. It was also clear that he could see that something was not quite right.

"Where are you going?" I asked her. "We need to stay; Jess is nearly finished."

"I need to go."

"Can you stay five minutes more?"

"No."

I said to the boss man, "I'm sorry, she is not well, we need to go. We can offer you $700, but you need to know, if she goes, I go with her and I have the money."

We walked away with the rug for $800 and one very happy son. The owner told us we got the deal of the year. Maybe it was the deal of the week, or the day, or the hour, but it made me happy believing him.

Alice

I did not take much, if any, notice of the wonderful history surrounding me that day. My mind was busy sorting voices and literally just putting one foot in front of the other. Holding Mum's hand seemed to keep me grounded but by the time we reached the carpet shop I was ready to leave.

I still had not pieced together that what I was experiencing was an illness, all I knew was that it was terribly frightening to be in the Bull, in Bardo, even with my family by my side.

Sarah

Sadly, the Blue Mosque, an icon of religious and architectural history, would have to wait for another trip as Jesse walked us back down through the maze of spice markets and out onto the road and put us in a cab. He then went off to wander around the old city, to soak up some of the history, knowing that under current circumstances it was all we would be able to sample.

The taxi driver that Alice and I travelled with had concluded that we were tourists and fair game for being ripped off. I gave clear directions by handing him the card with the hotel's address on it. He waved his hands in the air, proceeded to drive for about fifteen minutes down a few back streets, then onto a main road crowded with cars and then into a tunnel in the middle of which he stopped. Where he stopped looked like a large bus interchange and he told us we had to get out, he gesticulated in the direction of a light shining on a staircase. I pointed to the card sitting in his console with our address on it and he pointed to the door. When he showed me the fare, my mouth gaped open, but I was too tired to argue with where he had dropped us or care about the exorbitant cost. I paid and we went.

Considering my navigation skills are abysmal and Alice was no help at all, I then wondered how long it would take us to find our hotel. We walked up the dimly lit stairs and stepped out into the brilliant sunlight on a thriving tourist square. We moved further out into the middle of the square and I turned my face to the heavens. The sun was shining, the sky was the most beautiful blue and most importantly I had my girl right beside me.

I had much to be thankful for that day.

Alice with her music playing through Jesse's headset was oblivious to it all. I tugged her hand and pointed skywards and she lifted her head with her eyes closed and just let the sunshine down on her face. I watched as the slightest glimmer of a smile appeared, fleetingly, but when she opened her eyes and focused them on me for just a second and darted away, they were empty.

We moved to the edge of the square to try and find some landmark that I could locate on the tourist map. Then I asked Al if she was familiar with where we were and was surprised when she mumbled, "Yes, this way," and off we walked. We did the old walk-in-circles trick for about ten minutes before the penny dropped and I realised I was taking directions from a girl whose brain was not functioning and was perhaps shutting down. We stopped, still holding hands. I got my map out and tried to work out where the hell we were. Finally, after looking at the pictures on the tourist map, I figured out the way to the hotel, which turned out to be a thirty-minute meander back to the safety and familiarity of the hotel, which knowing my navigation skills, was a small miracle.

When I saw the hotel, I said a little 'woohoo' and punched my arm to the sky in joy and relief. This was only for me as Alice was in her own world. I couldn't get us in the door fast enough and we then both fell onto the bed, exhausted. I hoped that meant that we would sleep well that night.

Jesse returned about an hour or so later. Very pleased with his carpet purchase and the little bit of sight seeing that he was able to cram in without us.

***

Later that afternoon, Houssain came over with Rima and Batool, who were two more of Alice's wonderful Syrian friends who wanted to say goodbye before we left the next day.

They came up to our hotel room. Houssain introduced us and there were hugs all around. We sat in the chairs and on the end of Jesse's bed, which collapsed as if on cue, resulting in tears of laughter, which had been missing over the last week and were much needed natural medicine in the form of 'happy therapy'.

I had some English breakfast tea, delicious fresh Turkish baklava bought from the markets that morning and a large packet of chips to finish off our gourmet selection for afternoon tea.

Rima and Batool held Alice and hugged her, while Hossain kept a careful and protective eye on her. They told us how wonderful Alice was and how sad they were that she was going. While they were all talking, Alice laughed at something one of them said. Batool started crying, wiped her eyes and whispered to me that she had not seen Alice this animated for over a week. She was happy that her friend was going home, but sad that she would be losing her as well.

When it was time to go, they all cried, Jesse and I too. Alice had no tears, she seemed to be blank. She knew she should be sad, but it appeared that she couldn't find the emotion.

I took photos in the hotel room and out on the street before they left, the four musketeers. Then there were three …

Three of the most wonderful people I will ever have had the pleasure to meet.

After they left, I asked Alice if she was sad. She told me that she knew she should cry but the emotion for tears was just not there. It was like it had been switched off.

CHAPTER 13

Flashback

Monday 29 June 2015

Alice

The night of the full moon, my ability to hear voices was in overdrive. It was like I was in a giant pool where a ripple could change the tide at any second and sweep all the positive voices away with it. Everyone was commenting on Houssain and I. Our mismatched western–eastern relationship causing a schism in the tides. We arrived by the waterside and a giant ship rolled through the port in complete darkness. I interpreted this as a sign that I would be rescued and taken away by boat, back to Australia.

That night I had vivid dreams, one of these dreams involved a dark ship and a thunderstorm. Another delusion was birthed! That parasitic metaphysical beings had arrived via spaceships to sponge up the negative energy the world exudes. In that moment, it was even more important to focus on the positive voices, but on the walk to the water the negative voices were very alluring. It was hard to smile.

CHAPTER 14

Last day in the Bull

Wednesday 2 September 2015

Sarah

That final morning, I felt the need to express my sincere and heartfelt gratitude to Houssain and Alice's Syrian family. I spoke with Houssain but I needed him to know exactly how we felt, especially to acknowledge what they did to keep Alice safe and alive in the days preceding our arrival. The only problem was that I didn't have a nice card or any paper. The only alternative was to message him.

> *We would not have her if it were not for you. You are our little Syrian family and forever in our hearts. Hopefully one day we will all meet up again.*

Thank you, seems such a little word for the amazing thing you have done.
All our love and best wishes for the future to you and your wonderful friends.
Ba Sim
Batool
Kholod
Rima
Manar
You, of course, and anyone that I have missed.
Please give them a huge hug and kiss from my family, for all that each of you have done for her. Every bit of love and concern has helped and is aiding her to pull herself out of this 'depression' or whatever it is.
She will get there, I know.
She will miss you all.

Houssain's simple response amazed me. Alice had been so very blessed to have met him.

I have done nothing unusual; I love this girl and would do anything for her.

I was so very grateful for the day the sun shone on Alice and Houssain meeting.

Our night's sleep was much the same as the night before, though Alice at least did not try to leave the apartment. Her sleep was restless and filled with nightmares so she was grumpy and not seeing much sense on our returning to Australia and going to the doctors or to hospital when we got home.

She was confusing fact and fiction.

Alice still thought the bombs were going off. We kept reiterating that the loud noises were the music from the same night club a few streets away.

The one positive thing was that within twenty-four hours, she was at least speaking and not whispering or mumbling. She had words and we could try and make some sense of what they meant by delving through the fiction to find the truth.

There were moments that she was aware that her mind was playing tricks on her, but mostly she was living in a world of confusion and delusion.

Our taxi was booked for 9 am as we were not exactly sure how long it would take for us to get from Taksim Square to Atatürk Airport. Hopefully leaving early would give us plenty of time to get to our plane, which was scheduled to depart at 13:30, but also not so early that we might lose Alice, literally or figuratively.

We spoke with Alice and discussed the plan for the morning and tried to cover all our bases and explain everything to her. The taxi, the drive, the airport, the crowds, the plane trip. This information was repeated to her several times, but we needed to try and move her into reality with some sort of knowledge of what was to come. Our urgency to leave Turkey behind would need Alice to be on her best behaviour. Smoke and mirrors.

Houssain and Kholod arrived early for coffee. To see Alice, as it could be the last time they would see her for a very long time, if ever again.

As we said our goodbyes in the apartment, I tried to give these most wonderful humans some money. I had thought of a dozen ways of how to do it with the least embarrassment involved, but at the end of the day the only way to do it was to just give it to Houssain. I put it in an envelope so as not to embarrass them anymore.

Of course, they would not accept it.

"Alice has been staying with you for nearly a month, living with you and eating your food," I said. "Please take this money." I could see that they had very little.

"No."

"Please, think of it as rent money."

"No."

"Take it and spend it on whatever you want for all of you, please."

And finally, "No, it is not our way."

I approached Kholod and the answer was the same. No.

In hindsight I should have put it in a card and told them to read the card after we had gone, the problem would have been solved.

We left the hotel room with bags in tow, took the tiny lift two-by-two, like animals leaving Noah's Ark, then went out onto the street to await the taxi.

It amazes me what a hug can express. None of us wanted to let go. I wondered *if* in fact we would ever see these most magnificent humans again.

Jesse, Kholod and I stepped to the side and let Alice and Houssain have a private moment. I could not help but look as Houssain held

Alice's face between his palms and spoke quietly to her. She nodded and they embraced tightly, so tightly, like they never wanted to let go. They kissed and hugged again, and she turned to us. We silently walked her to the car, leaving those wonderful people behind, crying.

Our girl was too distressed and could not look back. We all cried. She held my hand ever so tightly and the tears she did not think would fall, finally, rolled down her cheeks. I gently wiped them away, leaving her in the moment. I felt so sad for her and what had happened, but ever so grateful to those that helped save her.

Alice

On the way to the airport in the taxi I could not bear to see what we were going past. I felt that if I saw anything, I would be telling the bad people that we were going to the airport, further putting my family in danger. I put my head in Mum's lap and shut my eyes, scared that our cab would be stopped, and we would never be let out of the Bull. The thought of being stuck there terrified me.

Sarah

Alice held my hand, squeezing it so tightly that I had to gently loosen her fingers. In return I gently squeezed hers, so she knew that I was there. She had her headphones on with her calming music, loud enough to help ease the cacophony of sounds and voices going on in her head. I noticed her eyes were squeezed shut and her free hand was shielding them.

Heading away from our hotel near Taksim Square, we drove

across the Galata Bridge spanning the Golden Horn of Istanbul, farewelling the crowds of tourists, the swirling fusion of people who lived there and what little of Istanbul we had seen. We caught a glimpse of the Blue Mosque on our right and the Bosporus on our left. We were leaving our Syrian family behind and wishing that we could bring them with us, or at the very least see them safely settled somewhere that they could call home.

The taxi driver was kind enough to point out a few of the ancient buildings on our way. Jesse was treated to a history lesson and soaked it up, but to be honest I was not listening. Alice was trapped in her own world and that was all that mattered to me. Dreaming through millennia of history, my only care was my daughter, Alice, and her safe travel to home, to care, to recovery and to the future.

CHAPTER 15

Airport chaos

Wednesday 2 September 2015, 11:30 am

Sarah

Around forty-eight hours after we first arrived in Istanbul, we were back at the airport to start our journey home. It was a bustling place of chaos and activity. That was the situation we were the most concerned about; how Alice would respond in the unfamiliar environment. Jesse and I were deeply concerned at the markets, but we were on red alert at the airport.

Jesse

We had one last step to go, to get Alice home. This meant we had to navigate the quagmire of Atatürk Airport and get her onto the plane. With Alice's impulsivity alone, getting her through the security and crowds was going to be difficult. In an attempt to make it as easy as possible to get us all through security and immigration, then onto the plane, we arrived a half hour earlier than the boarding desks opened, to be first in the queue, orientate ourselves, sort out a plan to get through the airport and preferably to wait for the flight in a quiet airport lounge.

When we arrived it immediately became clear that, no matter the planning, it was going to be a trying time getting through security to the quiet tranquillity of a lounge. We told Alice that she was not to go anywhere by herself, not to the bathroom or to sit alone. Not that she could, as Mum hadn't let go of her hand since she had tried to run away after we had left Houssain's apartment on the day that we had arrived.

The day before there had been a terrorist scare somewhere in the country and security was tight, meaning the lines were long. And I mean *long*. Long enough to make it touch-and-go to get to your flight's gate in time, even if you arrived three hours early like us!

The main issue was the line to get through the initial boarding check. The only real way to describe it is chaos. The line snaked and folded in on itself more than ten times and was about thirty metres long in each fold of the snake. It would take us about two hours to get through the queue. With Alice as she was, I agreed wholeheartedly with the assumption of her friends days earlier, that there was no way she was going to last through that line without an international event. It was going to be hard to do this with both the language barrier and the fact that no one could skip the line.

It was time to pull on some heart strings. I had already had a brief chat with a woman who was supervising the airline staff and first-class line, which ultimately skipped security entirely. I had worked out that we were not eligible for entry through that gate via the normal means. A quick chat with Mum and Alice and we were going to have to rely on the people staffing the gate seeing that it was important to let us through swiftly because we truly did have an unwell passenger to mind through the airport.

It was the same attendant who I had spoken to earlier. I indicated to her the loud and noisy line that we both knew would take hours. I implored her with my eyes to see that Alice was not going to do well in that line. *Just look at her, she can't do this right now*, I said in my mind. "She is not well," I said out loud. Mum was holding Alice's hand, looking just as trapped as Alice. I was the inmate grasping the bars and pleading our innocence. The attendant was a guard with a heart and, more importantly, a guard with the empathetic sense to feel what we were telling her.

Sarah

My heart pounded as we walked over to the first-class and business-class passport control check and Nearly-doc took control.

He spoke to the woman whose job it was to make sure any riff-raff like us did not jump the queue. Jesse had his long hair tied in a man bun, stubble from four days on the road adorned his face and he carried a hippie backpack. With a look of weary determination on his face, he calmly explained that he had travelled to Turkey with his mother to bring home her ill daughter and his sister.

There was no way, he told her, pointing to the queue, that we could take her through that, then he gestured at Alice and pointed to the economy and passport control line.

I hoped that this lady hadn't noticed the dark tentacles wrapped tightly around Alice's body, because if she did, she surely would not have let us through.

She looked at us and held her finger up in the air, gesturing to another official and Jesse explained the situation again. My heart was pounding. The woman spoke quietly to the other official and looked at us, at Alice, at Jesse and back to Alice and motioned us through. As we passed them, I grasped the lady's hand with tears in my eyes and said, "Thank you." Even now, writing this brings tears down my face. What was probably a very simple decision for her was a momentous one for us.

One crisis averted and we were one step closer to home. What we will never know is if waiting in that line would have caused problems, but we can only assume that being in such a confined space with so many people around would have had a disastrous effect on everything already going on in Alice's swirling brain.

We went through passport control and Jesse made us stop to look back at the horrendous line we had avoided. I hugged Jesse and could not help but do a little happy dance, which brought a confused look from Alice and a wry grin and a shake of the head from Jesse.

Now we just needed to get on the plane.

I had looked online and booked and paid for us to enter a lounge. We needed to remove ourselves from the mayhem of the terminal, another great idea of Jesse's that benefited us all and decreased our stress levels. I could take Alice to the bathroom and not worry that she would disappear, we could eat food, charge our phones, or in Alice's case stare vacantly into the distance.

Soon we would have travelled 28,000 kilometres in seventy-two hours to bring our precious girl home to start her recovery.

To board our plane, one of the factors that we had not considered was that we would be standing in an overcrowded airport bus that meandered around the huge airport for about twenty-five minutes to get to where our plane was waiting. Jesse and I flanked Alice and tried to be a buffer between her and other people.

When we arrived at the plane, Jesse reminded Alice about how when they left a country on their Roads Less Travelled Tour, they would kiss the ground when they arrived and then again on departure. So, before we headed up the stairs to board the plane, much to the amusement of the other travellers, they got on their knees and did exactly that. It seemed like they had both come full circle and it was time to start anew. I hoped for Alice that that was true.

Once aboard and in our seats, we turned our phones off and adjusted our seatbelts and tightened them for all it was worth. We knew this would be one roller coaster of a ride.

The leg from Istanbul to Singapore seemed to go on forever. Other than a few micro naps, neither Alice nor I could sleep. We had three seats together in economy and we are all fairly tall, so we felt like sardines squished into a can. At least I could watch the in-flight entertainment to keep myself occupied, but Alice's brain could not cope with that, so all she had was her wandering mind and the music that played continually in her ears via Jesse's headphones.

Before we left Istanbul, we had a discussion regarding when we should let Alice's good friends know a little of what had happened. To us it seemed that there is such a negative stigma that goes with mental health that we were conflicted as to whether to inform them. So, after much discussion, we decided to send out a text to a select few friends hoping that Alice would get the love, support, strength, and friendship that she needed.

Shane, Jess, and I agreed that the sooner her closest friends knew, the better. She would need them to band around her, to be her network, reassure her and inspire her in the weeks and months to come.

While on the plane to Istanbul, I had looked backwards in time to try and identify any red flags that I had missed about Alice. On the flight home to Sydney, it was time to reflect on my role as a parent. To consider the hard questions, whether I had contributed somehow to Alice's current mental health crisis.

As a parent, I know there are times when I have definitely dropped the parenting ball. I needed to look inward to see what that was so I could become a better parent and human.

Love, nurture, teach right from wrong, lead by example.

I am the first to admit that I was a better mother with our youngest child, Harry. Alice was eight years old and Jesse was eleven when Harry was born. We would call him our 'blessing baby' because so many of our friends would say, "Was he unplanned?" He may have been exactly that but we never wanted him to think he was unwanted!

When Jesse and Alice were kids, I was constantly tired and grumpy. This resulted in lots of yelling and tears, me as well as the kids.

I used to say that I woke up like Julie Andrews (the actress in *The Sound of Music*) and thirty minutes later I would turn into Cruella de Vil (from *101 Dalmations*).

By the time Harry came along, I knew that I could do better. I also had two wonderful helpers that adored their new little brother.

I guess we muddled along. There was more structure, the older two were at primary school and becoming their own little human beings and it was a joy watching them. I was still tired.

Alice was an accomplished swimmer and netballer. When she was thirteen, she wanted to stop competition swimming and training. The red flag was waving. I was sad and disappointed that she wanted to stop and I could not understand why. I can recall asking her and she said she just didn't want to do it anymore. I did not delve deeper. If I had I might have found the real answer.

What I learned years later was that she was being bullied incessantly by the girls in the swim squad about pimples on her back.

There is no way thirteen-year-old Alice would confront these girls. The so-called 'cool' kids of the swim club. They undermined her mentally and put a seed of anxiety and self-doubt in her that had not existed the year before. Where was I when this was happening?

I was there but not looking for the signs that were surely right in front of me. Lack of self-esteem, anger and a sadness seemed to permeate her being. This I can see was exacerbated by me not going in to fight for her at the swim school.

If I had talked to her more about the why, I am sure I could have made this time for her so much better, but I didn't. If I did learn the truth, what could I have done with this knowledge? I could have spoken with the swim coach and perhaps a plan of action could have been put in place. But at the very least she would have had our family support and strength behind her, rather than facing this bullying and belittling situation silently and alone.

Around this time, I used to say, "The hormones are strong in Alice." What I think now is that it was mental ill health knocking on the door.

Over the next few years Alice and I had a relationship of yelling at each other. With me being angry at her for something stupid, the clothes she wore or the way she spoke to me. I actually have a saying now: "Is it worth it?"

"Does it matter that they're wearing Ugg boots out or their hair needs a wash? Is it worth it? Is it hurting anyone? No. So don't stress over it!"

I did not listen to her or ask enough questions. I did not hear what she was saying because I didn't take the time and have those special moments that we should have had.

There are a lot of would-haves in these last few sentences. There are no woulda, shoulda, couldas in my vocabulary now. Hindsight is a most wonderful thing. If I can learn, move on and educate others from my own mistakes then I will take that as a positive.

I do not have a magic wand and hindsight cannot take me back in time.

Why do all these seemingly little things that I have mentioned matter? They matter because they hurt and are pieces of the puzzle.

When Alice's mental health was not great, I had no idea as she didn't confide in me, or maybe she simply did not think I would listen.

What have I learnt?

To listen. To love unconditionally. Although that can drive you to distraction, especially when you have to wade knee-deep through the floordrobe in their room.

I've learnt to be their parent first and foremost, not their best friend.

Perhaps the greatest gift to them is to be there for them when they make mistakes.

I have so much more to learn about being a parent. I guess you never stop.

Once we disembarked from the plane, it would be home to Shane and Harry. The next day, Alice would be evaluated by a doctor. We would all be able to start to heal. With my big girl pants pulled up high, I thought to myself, *We've got this.*

CHAPTER 16

Home

Thursday 3 September 2015

Sarah

The flight from Singapore to Sydney was uneventful, the only distress being that I was worried. In fact, I had worried the entire time we were away so I guess there was no change there! None of us slept. It was the theme of the last few days on repeat. Alice spent the time listening to music and the terrifying voices in her head and it was Jesse's and my job to be her mind guards. To redirect, when necessary, to skip a song, to help her eat or escort her to and from the bathroom. The seemingly insignificant act of eating the airline food was beyond her. She would look at the meal tray with confusion. This required Jesse or me to remove the foil from the dinner plate, butter her bread, shake the salt and pepper out of the wrappers onto her food and peel the top from her juice drink. Then hand her cutlery to her and tell her to eat.

We arrived back in Sydney where Shane and Harry met us at the airport. They were overjoyed to see us but even more so, they were eager to see exactly how Alice was with their own eyes. The greatest joy though was to have her back. They saw an Alice that was outwardly the same. The same one that left on her holidays a few months ago. The inner Alice was changed forever.

We had managed to get her home. Now the next part, the hardest part, was going to be getting an actual diagnosis and starting her recovery.

Alice

The minute I breathed in Australia's fresh air I felt like I was out of the Bardo and things were finally, nearly, almost back to normal. On the drive home from Sydney Airport, I could still feel a strong over-the-top interconnectivity with everything and an exaggeration of events' meanings. When we got home, birds flying around the house, for example, would mean that the thoughts I was having were acceptable. Cars beeping would mean for me to stop my chain of thoughts. Surprisingly, I had no idea that my mental health was so bad.

Why I was back home in Australia was a mystery to me, I came home simply because Mum and Jesse told me that was what we were doing.

There were so many voices in my head that all I knew was that if I was going to listen to any voices, it should be theirs and that I should trust them.

Sarah

It was early evening and we were exhausted but so happy to be back, at least Jess and I were. We were unsure of what Alice was thinking. At the dinner table a few short hours after we returned, we saw another example how Alice had absolutely no understanding of how ill she was. We talked about going to see our local doctor the next day and she was irritated as to why she needed to go and was confused about why we were even suggesting it. I did not have the energy to engage in a discussion and let the conversation move in another direction.

Shane saw for the first time the strong grip those dark tentacles had on our girl. Alice was looking at the television and telling us there was negative energy filling the room and we must get crystals. Shane looked at me in bewilderment. I shrugged my shoulders, raised my eyebrows, and realised just how happy I was to be home. A problem shared is a problem not solved in this case but at least halved.

When we headed to bed, I was still concerned that she might wander in the night and forget where she was, so I slept with her. I had asked Shane to deadlock all the doors, so if Alice tried to leave, it would be nearly impossible.

For insurance, we locked car keys, sharp knives, razors and drugs, in fact anything that could cause harm, in a cupboard. We only took the obvious, it would have been too hard to strip the house of everything harmful. At one stage we had too much to fit in our little locked cupboard, so I put it in the next best place – where I had hidden the Xbox years before when the kids' behaviour became obnoxious. Where, you ask? In the boot of the car, wrapped up in a shopping bag. The kids would go through the house looking everywhere for it and never, ever suspected the car.

Dastardly brilliant and, yes, you are welcome for the tip.

***

My sleep was disrupted by Alice waking several times, once to get up and go for a walk, who knows where to. Thankfully, I convinced her to come back to bed. I held her hand and stroked her forehead, just like I did in Istanbul, and I flashbacked to twenty-one years earlier when she was a baby. I would pick her up and cradle her in my arms, smell her sweet baby smell and stroke her little head to get her to sleep.

When we were trying to get back to sleep, she sat bolt upright and said "Mum, why is Turkish money like it is?" and "If a bird is in a cage, how do you get it to live out of a cage?" After a few seconds when my heart rate had decreased. I said, "These are amazing questions Alice, both of which I do not know the answer. Let me sleep on it." Any excuse at that moment, as my poor tired brain could not think of anything useful to share.

We finally fell into some sort of sleep. She woke up at one point moaning and mumbling gibberish. When I asked what was happening, she couldn't tell me in words what was going on in that chaotic mind of hers.

I prayed for morning.

Reality was blurry to her. Her mind was playing tricks and the voices made it difficult for Alice to be in the here and now. An example of this was when we were driving to the local doctor the next day and Jess and I started talking about the only dinner we had out in Istanbul and Alice said, "What about all the shit they put on our table."

"What shit, Al?"

"Seriously Mum! All the poo they dumped on our table was disgusting, I wanted to walk away but you wouldn't let me, then we just sat there with it, and ate our dinner!"

The restaurant was clean and so was our table, I recalled Alice had mumbled and stood up to leave at one stage. We had made her stay. Now it became clear as to why she had got up to leave in such an agitated state. She thought we could see and hear exactly what she saw and heard.

For her to stay sitting that night at a table with a pile of poop on it was a miracle and I can only assume a testament to her belief in us.

CHAPTER 17

Doctors, doctors, doctors

Friday 4 September 2015

Sarah

Alice was happy for Jess and I to go into her consultation with the doctor. In truth, I doubt if she would have known what to say. When the doctor enquired as to how she was, she said she was fine, that she was unsure what all the fuss was about and wondered why she was actually there. After hearing Alice recount her reason for returning home, the doctor thought Alice should make an appointment with a psychologist. Jess and I listened in, and my eyebrows shot up to the ceiling at the suggestion a psychologist would be the next step. If we were not there, I have no doubt Alice would have left the appointment with the doctor being none the wiser about the true state of her mental health.

I asked that doctor if it was okay, with Alice's consent, if Nearly-doc could talk about what occurred in Istanbul and what it took to bring Alice back home. After this new information Jesse provided, the doctor asked Alice some more questions. She followed up by saying, she thought it would be a good idea to go straight to the emergency department, to be seen by the psychiatric team in order to be assessed and perhaps admitted to hospital.

When we got back in the car, Alice was annoyed and angry that she needed to go to hospital. She believed that it was a waste of time and energy. She thought she could get better at home and she did not need anyone to help her. We had discussed with Alice before we got to the doctors about what might happen, and that the most likely scenario would be that she would be admitted to hospital. Clearly, she did not understand the conversation, or perhaps her mind had taken her off to a different place.

We arrived at the hospital to an empty emergency department. It was 9:30 on a Friday morning and normally the emergency department is mayhem at that hour. Luck was on our side so far.

Within five minutes, all her vital signs were checked, and her general history provided, for the **first** time to the triage nurse. Blood was taken and ten minutes later she was in a hospital gown, lying on a trolley bed in triage. It was there that the initial assessment was done before they moved her into a hospital bed in the accident and emergency ward. That room was large enough for twenty patients, with brightly striped curtains that could be pulled around each bed for some visual privacy only. In the centre was office space for the nurses and doctors to work on their notes, order tests, sort their paperwork and look at their patients.

Not long after, the Accident & Emergency registrar took her general history, for the **second** time, and read through the information that her brother had recorded in Istanbul.

"Invaluable," he said to the soon-to-be-doctor. We (actually just Alice, but it felt like Jess and me, too) were then transferred into the emergency ward with the same design of interior as the previous room. The emergency nurse then went through Alice's history for the **third** time.

The mental health nurse arrived, and Alice was whisked away to a private room to be further evaluated and assessed, and yet another history was taken, for the **fourth** time.

Meanwhile, Jess lounged on Alice's bed and I sat beside him on one of those hard uncomfortable chairs.

He wondered whether anyone would notice if he curled up on Alice's bed as jet lag had reared its head with that *must sleep* imperative.

An hour later Alice returned, just as the psychiatric registrar arrived. We left to have lunch and for Alice to be interrogated, oops interviewed, for the **fifth** time in three hours. By now, our girl had had it. She was exhausted and over everything, especially the part about being in hospital and answering the same questions repeatedly.

When we returned, it was our turn to be interviewed by the psychiatric registrar.

We left Alice in her bed, no one was with her. There were probably ten other patients and six staff monitoring their health but surely not their whereabouts. I worried that she would not be there upon our return and hoped that someone was keeping a close eye on her. Even though I am familiar with medical settings, the fear and vulnerability of this sort of crisis sets one's nerves on edge.

The psychiatric registrar began by asking us a few questions. Nearly-doc Jess explained that he had taken a full history from her friends in Istanbul and handed his iPad over for her to read.

"Would you like a job? This is brilliant," she said.

When we finished, the psychiatric registrar was armed with the information and headed off to share her knowledge and observations of Alice to the big doctor guy, her boss. No diagnosis had been made yet.

We returned to Alice, who was surprisingly still sitting in her bed, we waited there too. I need not have worried about anyone keeping a close watch on her. Fortunately for us, she was on WhatsApp with Houssain. He was keeping her grounded for the moment and listened to all her delusions without passing judgement.

The registrar returned and told Alice they were going to treat her for a drug-induced psychosis. She needed to be admitted, started on antipsychotic medication, and needed an EEG (electroencephalogram, it tracks and records brain waves) and a CT scan of her brain, to rule out any underlying cause, like a brain tumour. Last and by no means least, she was to be scheduled under the Mental Health Act, which meant that she could not discharge herself from the hospital, only a doctor could release her. That meant that at that stage of her illness, she was a threat to herself and could not make the best decisions for herself.

My heart broke for my girl.

Alice, of course, did not agree with the decision and only heard the doctor say that she needed to stay in hospital. Our day had started at 8 am and it was after 3 pm when we all got that news from the registrar.

I texted Houssain with the update. That she had been admitted to hospital, that she was not happy about it, and that she would start medication later that night. He responded.

I am trying not to worry. Honestly, knowing that she is in the hospital now just broke my heart, though I had this possibility in my mind.

CHAPTER 18

White walls

Friday 4 September 2015

Sarah

Seven hours after we arrived at the hospital, Alice had a confirmed bed in the short-stay psychiatric ward – the Psychiatric Emergency Care Centre, or PECC unit. It was a six-bed mental health unit at our local public hospital. We had no idea what awaited us, but I had the positive visions of nurses coming to greet us with warm smiles and hugs.

We walked there together down a maze of corridors with white walls featuring an assortment of printed artworks. Into the lift and then along more corridors, a bit like snakes and ladders; Jess, Alice, a transfer nurse, an orderly and me. We knew we had arrived when we came to a double set of locked doors. To enter, we needed to use the intercom to be buzzed through the first door.

Briskly the nurse hustled Alice through the second lot of doors. Before we relatives were allowed through the next set of doors, we were given a locker where we placed any handbags, backpack, shoelaces, belts, plastic bags, phones or other electronic devices in our possession. The risk of suicide and self-harm must sadly be ever present in that locked ward.

Finally, we went through the second set of doors and were greeted by white walls, a smattering of green plastic plants and a neutral environment.

Alice's room was huge, you could have fit two beds easily but there was only one (on wheels that were locked), as well as a simple bedside table and a chair with that pseudo-soft padding on it. Cold, empty and sterile. Sadly, it was exactly what I thought a stereotypical room would look like in a psychiatric ward. A light switch was beside the door, which had a lock on the outside.

I felt like crying, again.

I felt depressed and I was not even the one that had to stay there.

Alice was unable to comprehend that her room in this locked ward was the best place for her at that moment. She thought we were deserting her. The medical staff had not quite realised her exhaustion was due not only to the psychosis but to her jet lag as well. We all agreed that she still did not understand or realise how sick she was.

When we left Alice, I turned back to watch her. Over her shoulders and wrapped around them were the dark tentacles of mental ill health, squeezing her ever so tightly.

A few hours after Jesse and I left the ward, a low dose antipsychotic tablet was given to her. Jesse had said the saying is 'go low, go slow'. Start off with a low dose and see how the patient does, because that may be the perfect dose for them. If not, the dosage is increased until you get to the correct level, or you start all over again with a different drug. I liked it. Alice did not. In the meantime, the nurses came in and asked her yet another round of questions. This made it the **seventh** time that she had been interviewed in as many hours.

***

We found the recounting of a medical history seven times extremely frustrating but the medical personnel were, in truth, on a fact-finding mission so to speak. Her medical history was documented directly from Alice, Jesse or me. This cut out the middle person and the chance for any medical evidence to be misconstrued or distorted. Like in the game 'telephone' where a chain of people whisper a phrase to the next person. By the time it comes out the other end it is completely different to how it started.

***

The next two days were much the same since nothing much happens on the psychiatric ward on the weekend. The nurses who were on that day did not go and sit and chat with her. The enclosed office area was raised up a step with a glass window. The thick emergency type. I imagine it can withstand chairs being thrown at it and would work as a refuge if a patient loses control and the staff need to retreat to safety. The glass surrounded three sides so there was an uninterrupted view of their patients.

The staff were typing on their computers or chatting among themselves while their patients watched television, read a book, a magazine, stared aimlessly into nothingness or looked at the small amount of green foliage in the tiniest of courtyards outside the window.

I had an overwhelming feeling of loneliness for Alice, and for me. I had an enormous bag of guilt and sadness hanging from my shoulder from the very fact that she was in there. And that bag was heavy.

Shane and I went to visit twice on the Saturday.

We arrived at the start of visiting hours to find Alice in bed asleep. She had had her breakfast and retreated. The antipsychotic drug, although much needed, had left our girl sleepy and extremely irritated. You could say the morning had not been kind. We didn't stay long as she could barely put two words together and was angry with us that she was in hospital, adamant that she did not need to be.

When we went back in the evening, we continued to have our animated discussion regarding the necessity of her being in hospital. Again, she could understand that she was ill, but there was nothing to see, no cancer to cut out, no bone to mend, no cut to suture and no rash to fix.

Her injury was unseen, yet no less life threatening.

It was heartbreaking to see her like this.

We needed to remember, an immediate cure or quick fix was extremely unlikely. Time and patience was what we needed, and we had plenty of that.

From *Dear Psychosis*,

I have seen the darkness.

I have felt the anger.

I have touched the sadness.

I have grieved what was lost.

I have cried over the unfairness.

I have succumbed to the silence.

I will not speak.

CHAPTER 19

Father's Day

Sunday 6 September 2015

Sarah

We were visiting more for us than for her, as at that moment in time she really could not care less if we were there or not. She was wrapped up in a world of eating, sleeping, taking her medications and then repeating.

Her world was a world of delusion. We were desperate to see when the antipsychotic medication would start making a difference. *Could it be today?* No one had given us any indication of anything really.

It was Father's Day and we were off to my brother's to join my extended family. There would be around twenty people there. I was anxious and, to be honest, I was a nervous wreck.

I thought time out of the house and seeing my family meant time away from our concerns and stress, but as we got closer to our destination, the more emotional I became.

They are my flesh and blood. I should be able to speak about what has happened. But I was scared. I just didn't want to impart anything that might label Alice. I was having difficulty knowing what was going on in Alice's brain, let alone being able to explain it to others. My immediate concern was people judging or coming to their own conclusions on what and how this had happened to Alice.

Psychosis is hard enough to explain to people, let alone a drug-induced psychosis.

The simple fact was we had no answers and were unlikely to have any for some time.

I should have realised that my family would be there for us, but I could not see through my grief as it was all too consuming.

I wish I had been able to express that in words to them all.

Looking back, I recognise that all my energy and focus was on Alice and getting her well – finding the correct medical team and looking for answers was our foremost concern.

I had confided in Shane, Jesse and to a certain extent little Harry and my sister Jane about what had happened. This was actually the case for the next few years. I had talked briefly with my darling parents. I was so emotional and raw regarding Alice's mental health. I could not find it in myself to truly share my grief and sadness with anyone. Shane had been my rock and had spoken to the rest of our families and told them what we knew, which was not much.

I hoped they understood my unwillingness to talk would not be forever. I wanted to say, *Don't give up on Alice and us.*

All I hoped for that day was that they would not ask me anything. At that stage I was incapable of sharing. I was certain that Shane felt very similar emotions but at this stage he was the strong one and I needed to lean on him. With all this in mind, Shane, Jesse, Harry and I walked into lunch late and within a minute someone said something innocuous, like 'Happy Father's Day' and the floodgates opened and I was crying.

The roller-coaster ride of the last week came back to me at full tilt with a sudden and crushing emotional explosion.

My brother and his wife did not know what to do. There were probably eight people in the lounge room, five of whom had a vague idea of what had happened. Their eyes darted from person to person as the message had been not to say anything. So, they didn't. I was immediately enveloped in Jesse's and my sister Jane's arms, with my brother-in-law, Mark, making soothing sounds behind me. I know they were confused and sad for us all too.

I was uncomfortable because I knew I had led and fed this feeling of palpable awkwardness.

They were not sure what they should be doing or feeling because they were not exactly sure what had happened in any sort of detail.

I was heartbroken and it was showing.

I knew that we were some of the lucky ones, we still had our beautiful girl with us. I could touch and feel her. Many others don't get that chance, in this we were blessed. There were others in a far worse situation.

It was the unknown of what Alice and we, as a family, were facing and what her life would be like in the future that was really upsetting me. I wish I could have articulated those exact words to my family.

I pulled myself together and wished I could have made some stupid joke, but I had nothing left to give. This time it was the cloak of sadness wrapped tightly around me.

I took a big breath, gratefully accepted a glass of wine, a big one, and went to sit at the table for lunch with red-rimmed eyes and a red nose.

I pretended that nothing had happened and everyone else joined in on the game and we played happy families for the next few hours.

The rest of lunch went to plan, and NO ONE asked me anything. I could only imagine how hard and confusing that must have been for them, especially those who were not aware of the events of the last week.

Our huge sigh of relief when we left was enormous. I can only imagine how my family felt.

When we got in the car, we talked about pretence, lying or, better yet, distorting the truth and putting up a facade. Why was it so hard for me to let people know what had happened?

I suspected for my part, at that time, mental health was a subject so open to debate. It is no wonder that people and their families do not 'come out' about their loved ones when there is so much judgement passed.

What does she have, what does it do, how does it affect her?

A drug-induced psychosis, what drug did she take?
Is she still taking drugs?
Does she take her medications?
Can she work?
Does she have a job?
Why isn't she working?

These are the questions we would be asked hundreds of times in the following years. Often by the same people every time we met up. They didn't ask those questions to be rude. They asked because they simply forgot.

That evening we drove Nearly-doc to the airport to fly home to Melbourne. Back to his studies, his girlfriend and his normal, everyday life. God, what would we have done without him that week? With a hug, a backpack full of love and a Turkish hall runner under his arm, Jess was gone.

We headed back to the hospital with Harry, it was 7 pm.

In the last forty-eight hours Alice had been making plans to surf, further her university degree, travel the outback and help First Nations communities. Apparently, these sorts of never-ending plans are not unusual during psychosis. So, we were keen to see what else had been added to her ever-growing list of things to do since we'd last seen her.

When we arrived, we saw the same white walls and staff behind the glass partition, only coming out to take her vital signs, blood pressure and temperature, and daily observations. They then retreated behind the thick glass wall to tap, tap, tap on their computers. There were five patients on the ward that night.

Alice greeted us, sitting at a table and introducing us to a slightly older girl. Probably in her late twenties. The young lady left us after a few minutes of telling us a vivid tale, her story, her truth in that moment. She danced away and we were left with Alice who just saw a fellow woman, enjoying her company. She did not comprehend that her new friend was spouting nonsense. In fact, I wondered what the conversation was like between the two of them. I would have loved to be a fly on the wall for that one.

Our girl was talking some sense and had a calmness around her that had not been present since before we met her in Istanbul. Hubby, Harry and I looked at each other and felt a glimmer of hope, that was our first positive step forward.

We left with optimism in our hearts.

CHAPTER 20

Back home

Monday 7 September 2015

Sarah

It seemed like a dream that it was only seven short days since we had landed in Istanbul, thrust into the unknown. Just a week before, we would never have dreamt our lives would be uprooted by mental ill health. There was much we had to learn. I suspected patience might be the first thing.

Monday morning arrived and I was not surprised to get a phone call from Alice's psychiatric registrar to tell us that she and the Big Guy had talked with Alice. They thought it was reasonable for her to come home *if* the family was happy and they released her into our twenty-four-hour care. She was no longer scheduled; one more tiny step in the right direction.

Yes, we were happy that she could come home. What that meant was that one of us had to stay home from work with her until her health improved. For the moment that person was me.

I rang both my jobs and told them I would not be back for another few weeks. The support from the very tiny group of people I worked with in the operating theatres was heart-warming. A kind word here or short text message there, saying that they were around anytime that we needed them did not go unappreciated. Kourosh, Katherine, Vince, Patrick, Kevin and Lillyann. They showed my family nothing but kindness and support.

When Alice and I returned home from the hospital, waiting at the front door was the most enormous bunch of beautiful flowers from those work colleagues.

I said to Alice, "These are for you, this is for a fresh start, in fact a positive start to the week and here's cheers to new beginnings."

The sun was shining.

The antipsychotic medication she was given was called Olanzapine. The psychiatric registrar had explained that this drug was classed as an antipsychotic and mood stabiliser and sounded like the perfect medication for Alice.

She started on 7.5 mg but had increased to 10 mg to be taken at 9 pm.

At home, still locked up was anything that we perceived to be a danger. It was amazing how much ibuprofen and paracetamol had been scattered throughout the house, in handbags, bathroom drawers and kitchen cabinets. The sharp stuff only came out to prepare dinner and then went back into lock up for safekeeping.

Plastered on the wall above our home phone was a large laminated A4 sheet of paper. On it were three phone numbers in black permanent marker. The first one was the PECC psychiatric unit number. Below that was the emergency out of hour's number for psychiatric emergencies and lastly our Australian emergency number, 000, for ambulance, police or fire.

I was so sad when I was writing these out, which was for two reasons. First and foremost, for the safety of Alice and secondly for Harry.

Shane and I had a heartbreaking conversation with him regarding what the numbers meant. To spell it out.

"Harry, if you come home and find your sister in any sort of condition, whether it is confused, dangerous, frightening or, God forbid, dead. These are the numbers to ring." I cried after talking with him; what a burden to put on him.

Harry, on the other hand, had taken everything in his stride. It was his sister, and life goes on. "What's for afternoon tea, Mum?" he said afterwards as he walked out the door to play basketball with the other kids in the street.

I then wrote a to-do list and the first order of the day was to call Harry's school and speak with his main teacher to explain what had happened and was happening in Harry's home life. I asked them to keep a close eye on him at school. To let me know if anything, especially his behaviour, changed and asked them to please contact us immediately if it did.

***

Alice took her tablet at 9 pm and it knocked her out.

In the first few days after being released from hospital, the process of getting her out of bed would start at 10 am. I opened her door and gently rubbed her shoulders, which achieved nothing. Then I would say her name and get a groan or two. I'd then proceed to pushing her shoulders until I got some movement. I'd then wait thirty minutes and go in again, this time announcing myself loudly and open the curtains. This would be accompanied by loud groans and unintelligible words. I'd persist and finally, if I was lucky, by 2 pm she would get out of bed. She looked exhausted, flat, and vacant. She was still in her pyjamas, but at least she was out of her dark, curtain-enclosed bedroom.

This approach was not a success.

I learnt quickly, what we both needed was a routine.

I chose the time 9:30 am as when I would wake her. I knocked on the door, opened it while speaking loudly and raised the curtains to let the natural light stream into her room. She was angry to be woken this way, but I'd leave her knowing that I would be back to push her out of bed and into the shower soon enough.

Alice's brain could only focus for a few minutes at a time, reading books, watching television, drawing, doing puzzles. Anything that required concentrating was out of the question. The psychosis had injured her brain. The result of this was that she was bored, lonely, sad, and angry.

I wish I had thought to read to her. This would have been therapeutic for both of us. Whether it be a novel, poetry, or a magazine. So, my gift to you, dear reader, is to encourage you do what I did not – read; I have no doubt that it will soothe your soul as well as your loved one.

The only thing Alice could do well after Istanbul and the PECC Unit was sleep. That came with a huge drawback of voices and nightmares. When that happened in the dark of night she would come and tell us. By this, I mean I would wake to Alice standing, just standing, at our door or beside me, which was a frightening way to be woken. When I'd eventually pull my heart back into my chest and extract my fingernails from the ceiling, I would get up and take her back to bed. If she told me to stay, I would crawl into bed next to her and have a sleepover. My instinct was in overdrive to keep her safe, while I cried inside at what my darling girl was going through.

Television gave her a headache as it strained her brain trying to follow a storyline. The national news, or in fact any negative or distressing news, especially the war in Syria and the boat people leaving Turkey, put her anxiety into overdrive.

For six months we did not watch news or current affairs. The fear was that Alice would hear some terrible event from the day and this would lead to anger and delusion.

Salvation came still in the form of Jess's trusty headphones that he had kindly left with her.

By the late afternoon, her mood altered from grumpy to negativity and her thoughts were scattered. The voices were crowded in her head. The doctors' only advice was that if that happened to take her medication at an earlier time. We decide to move it to 6 pm, just before dinner.

***

Wednesday 9 September 2015

Two days after her public hospital discharge, Alice had a follow up appointment with a psychologist at the outpatient department of the public hospital. I went armed with questions for the psychiatric team that we needed answered.

Driving on medication?

Yes, she can, no problem there.

How long will she be on antipsychotic medication?

How long is a piece of string really, but at least two years, maybe five, maybe for life.

What if she wants to go out and usually takes her meds at 6 pm?

That is fine, she can take them when she gets home.

Should she be drinking alcohol?

If she can abstain then that would be great, *but* in saying that she is twenty-one years old, if she drinks, it's best not to drive due to the alcohol interacting with her medication and making her drowsy.

What about recreational drugs?

There is a high risk of relapse into psychosis, so this is a definite no.

What are the chances of a relapse?

Unknown, but if she is compliant in taking her medication and does not take any illegal substances then chances of psychosis are dramatically decreased.

Last night she appeared anxious about all the new technology, what do we do when this happens?

Listen to her and hear her concerns.

Is it better to be in the private or the public system?

That's entirely up to you.

At the Wednesday morning appointment, Alice's antipsychotic drug dosage was increased from 10 mg to 15 mg of Olanzapine. Psychiatrists prescribe medications, treat and diagnose the patient. Psychologists focus on talking and providing therapy to the patients. I am not sure who increased her medication, but I assumed they went to Alice's Big Guy or his psychiatric registrar.

We needed to have faith and trust in the system.

An appointment was made to see the psychiatric registrar the following day at the outpatient department of the public hospital. Not the Big Guy. In fact, we never saw him, ever. It is odd how it never once crossed our minds while she was being treated to ask to speak to the Big Guy!

***

Alice continued to be confused between fact and fiction. She would dream about something and think that it was real, and the delusion would colour her day. Arguing with someone in this state is pointless and only caused frustration on both sides.

That night, two of Alice's friends were coming over after dinner for a quick visit and to see how Alice was. This felt like a good idea in theory, but in hindsight a day visit would have been better.

At the dinner table minutes before they arrived, Alice started rambling about new technology and how scary it is. The beginning of the conversation started off very innocently and we were lulled into thinking that it was a normal conversation. We were excited. Then it came to an abrupt halt when she talked about how the television was listening in on us. She desperately needed quartz stones or other such things to combat the messages being sent through the television cables. She urgently needed to go to the new age shop a couple of suburbs away to browse their crystals and select some stones, as she felt it would make everything better. Not right, but it would improve the situation. Alice gave us directions to where these crystals would need to be placed. She showed us a spot on each side of the television. These would combat the signals that were being received. This was detailed explicitly by Alice and every placement had to be just right.

I gave a panicked look to Hubby. *What do we do?*

Then the doorbell went and her friends arrived.

We had not been able to address what had just happened.

What could we say to the words that came out of her mouth,

as they made no sense to us. There was no logic, but to Alice it was crystal clear.

While Alice's friends were with her, Shane and I had a frantic whispered conversation about what we should do about Alice's delusional thoughts over the television. By the time her friends left, we were no closer to a solution, other than to go with our gut. Which was the path of least resistance. Go with the flow and if she still needed to visit the crystal shop the next day then I would take her.

After her friends left, I could see that she was exhausted. I said we needed to find the tools for her to be able to tell us or her friends when she was anxious or uncertain of herself. I was not exactly sure what they might be, but we were determined to find them.

We were so in the dark that manoeuvring through it was tough and we kept bumping into things. Figuratively, we were opening the wrong doors and using keys that did not work. Shane, Harry and I talked about this, but not one of us had an answer about how to overcome any of these obstacles and it was difficult to know who to ask.

***

Thursday 10 September 2015

The next day, on an unusually cold spring morning, we headed to the crystal shop. To Alice's credit, it was a quaint little space filled with beautiful stones. The incense was a little overwhelming, actually a lot, but I could still breathe. Which was a positive. The cost of the stones surprised me, even for the little ones they were quite expensive. Alice sourced a few beautiful crystals, each with a tiny card explaining what the stone does. The most notable one was a beautiful black one called tourmaline. We got two, for protection against technology. They would be placed on either side of the television. The next was a small purple piece called obsidian, the main use is protection against negativity. This would be in her pocket. Amethyst was next and would go under her pillow and help again with negativity. Her last stone was a smooth black worry stone, with an indent in the middle where you could rub your thumb. She gave it to me, to help me worry less about her. My heart melted; she was aware of how concerned we were about her.

We might not have believed in the power of crystals, but we were certainly open to them if it gave Alice some peace. (And just quietly, us too.)

Three months before, she had been living her dream of traveling, seeing different cultures, experiencing a different way of life, and meeting new and wonderful people from diverse backgrounds from all around the world. Now she was under our care, on medications and not able to comprehend the full picture.

She was brave, courageous, and very strong.

She had spent the last five days as an outpatient. She had daily phone calls from a nurse from the mental health clinic checking in on her.

Depending on the time of day, her moods swung erratically from calm and reflective to angry at what the drugs were doing to her mind, body, and soul.

We felt lost every time the outbursts happened. She would talk extremely fast; it is called rapid pressure speech; we called them 'verbal grenades'. As a family, we still had no pointers on what to do or say when Al was feeling particularly low or having negative thoughts.

I was hyper-aware of her moods, which led me to affect a constantly happy and positive appearance. A permanent smile was on my face when I was around her. It was exceedingly draining. Most nights, I'd fall into bed absolutely exhausted, only to wake throughout the night listening for Alice or waking to find her at our bedroom door. Or at the foot of the bed, just standing there rocking from side to side, unsure of what to do as she couldn't sleep. I would suggest things to do to get back to sleep, like counting backwards from one hundred. But then I realised she was unable to concentrate for any length of time, so it was useless. She couldn't read, so she lay awake listening to the voices in her head until she put her headphones on and concentrated on her music. Which at that stage was still the only alternative to the sounds going on in her brain.

We did not argue back when the verbal grenades started to come our way. Which was often. When they did come, they were painful to listen to and often made no sense to us. We simply did not know what to do or say to make things right, because there was no right way.

These grenades could be anything from a memory in her childhood, to a perceived or real time in her life where she was upset that we did not help her. There is no doubt some of her grievances were valid and we acknowledged what we could. But it was the left-field anger from incidents years before, incidents that we have no memory of, that had us in the dilemma of what to say or do. The simple fact was that these incidents may have been minor to us but they were huge to her just as the delusions that she saw were real to her. The wrongs we did, no matter if they were real or imagined, needed to be accepted, acknowledged, and recognised.

The tentacles of mental ill health were slowly squeezing the essence out of who she was, and we didn't know how to stop it.

***

Friday 11 September 2015

Sarah

On her Friday morning appointment, Alice saw yet another psychologist. Moving forward, I hoped this would be her regular one! I found a chair against the wall and started reading a gossip magazine and waited for Alice's appointment to finish.

A few other people were sitting dispersed in the galley-like waiting room. There was a tiny kitchen area set up at one end with a hot water urn, tea, coffee, milk and some sweet biscuits. The television was on with no sound, but there were subtitles. While I was lamenting this situation, I heard the receptionist talking on the phone about a private facility at St Vincent's Hospital called USpace. My ears pricked up as I listened in. I immediately opened the notes section in my phone and typed Google USpace so I didn't forget.

The psychologist came out to the waiting area and asked me to join them for the last ten minutes of Alice's appointment to go over, with Alice's permission, her medication changes, (an anti-anxiety drug had been added), and so I could ask any questions. My only concern at that time was the different psychologists Alice was seeing and wondered when she would be allocated a permanent one. The mental health team, that consisted of the psychologist, the mental health nurse, and the nurse unit manager, talked about staff rosters; yes, it would happen, hopefully the following week. It was hard not to show my frustration. I knew that consistency was a huge key and yet in the heart of the hospital outpatient unit the nuts and bolts that held everything together were not under the guidance of the same builder or architect. If we were not under the one roof how would Alice survive this torrential downpour.

***

After her psychologist's appointment on Friday, we were at home having a cuppa at the kitchen table. Alice talked of her frustration and said that she would rather take her own life than be on the drugs that she had been prescribed. She had been on medication for a week and was putting on weight, a known side effect and a major concern for her. Not knowing what to say to these statements was unnerving. It was the first time I had heard her mention suicide and it shook me.

The most important thing was that I acknowledged her feelings. I stated the obvious and said that I didn't want her to do that. We chatted for a while, mostly a one-sided conversation on my part, throwing ideas or options out about what we could do together. Perhaps daily walks with our dog Minnie, watching what we ate, joining the gym. I could go with her. These were all met with dismissive annoyance. I retreated and suggested that if she had any ideas, to voice them. What followed was silence.

I took her hands in mine and held them tightly and said, "No matter what the voices tell you or if you are thinking bad thoughts, please come to me. You know Dad and I are always here for you. Do you hear me?"

We hugged and she went to lie down, our outing to the psychologist had been both physically and mentally tiring.

It was late in the afternoon when I got on the computer and typed in 'USpace'. It looked like a relatively new facility. Think modern youth hostel vibe. It was specifically for young adults aged between sixteen and thirty years.

My heart lightened a little.

It felt like the first step in the right direction since Alice had been released from the public hospital.

There was a catch. It's a private psychiatric care facility. We needed our private health fund to come to the party and cover her stay.

By the time I called USpace, it was after 5 pm on Friday. All the important people had gone home and that meant they wouldn't be back until Monday morning.

Thankfully, I talked with one of the registered nurses. I shared Alice's story and our concerns. I was given a name to speak to, a time to ring on Monday and, most importantly, she gave me hope.

The mental health phone calls from the outpatient psychiatric nurses to Alice continued over the weekend.

Her first Saturday at home was a good day, at least for us. I blame Saturday for lulling us into a false sense of security because Sunday was awful.

***

Sunday 12 September 2015

Sarah

It started out with good intentions. The day was glorious, the sun was shining, the sky was blue, there was a gentle breeze and not a cloud to be seen, but due to lack of foresight, there was definitely rough weather ahead.

Alice went on her first outing since coming home from Turkey to a local circus with her friend, Lozza. The thought had crossed my mind that I should go with them, but in truth what I was doing was thinking about myself and my wants. I just needed a few hours of peace and calm to myself, not realising that this was a crucial time. Remember, this was only our second week into psychosis and mental ill health. An inordinate amount of patience was required and needed. You know the saying, *this is a marathon not a sprint.*

She needed us to be her conscience, her wisdom, and her voice.

Of course, I should have gone as all I did was worry the entire afternoon until she returned. I waited nervously by the front door, watching for her return. As soon as I saw her getting dropped off,

I jumped into a chair in front of the television, pretending I didn't have a care in the world.

All my subterfuge went to waste because the moment Alice opened the door it was clear that the circus had not been a success. Hyper-stimulation, too many people, too much noise, in fact too much of everything. In conjunction with the voices that shouted and took over her mind, it was just far too crowded in her poor exhausted brain.

The tentacles are black with confusion and anger. Wrapped tightly all around her body.

Foresight would have been helpful but none of us thought about the negative. We only thought about Alice getting out of the house and being with someone other than family. Would it have helped if one of us went with her? Absolutely.

The verbal grenades were lobbed the moment she set eyes on us. It didn't stop.

We knew it wasn't our Alice.

She paced around the house several times before the water boiled and I could get a soothing cup of herbal tea ready for us both, well, mostly for me. She doesn't like tea all that much. We went upstairs to the balcony and sat, more to soak up the peace of the afternoon than anything else. I was with her just to be with her.

A few hours later at dinner she became extremely agitated about not doing yoga, even though she hadn't done it in five months. And she spoke about not being with friends, we think she was talking about her friends from Istanbul, but this was unclear, and then she complained that she was bored. The yoga aspect would be an ongoing theme through the next few weeks and months. There was no rational discussion that took place that night.

***

Monday 14 September 2015

Sarah

The new week arrived bleak and stormy, and we were at Alice's Monday morning appointment.

Don't ask, but yes, with yet a different psychologist.

I was not sure if Alice was frustrated by this or the fact that in her short appointment, they spent half of it looking up her medical history and reading what the previous psychologists had documented rather than talking to her.

I sat in the waiting area and tried not to dwell on her having to see yet another psychologist. I was asked again to come in at the end and if I had anything to add.

Alice's antipsychotic medication was increased again, this time to 17.5 mg of Olanzapine. I reminded myself what Jess had said regarding her medications, "Go low, go slow," I knew they were helping her, but the negative was that it made her sleep for at least eighteen hours a day.

I understood the need for her brain to rest and we needed to trust that these people caring for her, knew what they were doing.

It was at that visit that they told us to lock away our knives and all medications. Ten days too late as far as I was concerned, we had done it Day One.

On our return home, I called USpace and spoke with the nursing unit manager. She listened to our girl's story and was positive that USpace was the right fit.

The immediate relief I felt was wonderful and I called Shane to let him know. Happy tears reigned supreme that day.

Hallelujah.

Uspace had a bed available two days later, on Wednesday, but as a private facility, our health fund had to be able to cover the costs.

Thankfully, after the longest twenty-four hours, we received positive news from the health fund that the hospital was *GO*.

Alice still could not understand why she needed to be admitted. The voices and cacophony of sounds in her head remained; disordered thoughts, negative feelings and low self-esteem. The verbal grenades continued to be lobbed at Shane and Harry, but I was the one taking the heaviest blows simply because I was around her all day, every day.

We had many chats before she went in to USpace. I sat with her in her bedroom or outside in the backyard and watched her pace while she talked or stomped through the house. Most of what she said I could not understand.

We needed to remember that it was only ten days since we brought Alice home from Istanbul. In those ten days we needed to be encouraged by the improvements she had already shown, little by little. It was essential for us to remember that we were moving forward not backward.

The critical element in all of this was that she needed to go to USpace voluntarily. They would not keep her there against her will. If she didn't want to be admitted or wanted to leave, they couldn't make her stay. If she harmed herself or was suicidal, she would not be admitted. If either of those happened, she would have most likely been scheduled and transferred to the psychiatric unit at St Vincent's Hospital. *Breathe*.

CHAPTER 21

USpace

Wednesday 16 September 2015

Sarah

I felt immense guilt that Alice was being admitted to hospital but at the same time I experienced deep relief. I would sleep better knowing that she was under the care of an experienced medical team who would watch her diligently. Harry would be able to walk around the house without stepping on eggshells. Shane would get a break from my numerous daily texts, which were hourly if I am honest. Most importantly I could go back to work. I could keep my mind occupied with mundane thoughts and our lives could return to some sort of order.

Was it normal that my emotions were entwined so confusingly? Were we being selfish?

What was best for Alice and at the same time what was best for Shane and me?

Shane and I questioned and double guessed everything we did. Mental ill health was not on our radar. We had been advised by the psychiatric registrar at the public hospital that Alice's psychosis may be a cover for a further mental health diagnosis, which increased our anxiety. We had heard stories on the news about psychosis but no one we knew had been down this road. That was how limited our knowledge was. We needed help, we just didn't know *who* to go to.

What we did know was Alice needed to be admitted as she wasn't safe at home. Her medications needed to be assessed and she needed to be under the care of a psychiatrist that was going to be regularly available to her. We hoped that that would bring routine and stability back into her life, and to ours too.

We were told to get to the hospital at 9 am, which meant enduring peak hour traffic in the car for an hour. The conversation on the way there was not scintillating, in fact the main topic was just: *why*.

"Because it is the right way forward for you to get better."

"But why?"

"This is where you need to trust us. I have no answers for you yet, but hopefully by staying there we can find some."

We checked in and waited for over an hour in the hospital admissions area to be admitted. We made sure to find seats with the least foot traffic going past. Sadly, that didn't stop the general clang and clatter of a hospital going on around us and we hoped that

Alice and her voices would stay with us.

The headphones with the tap to move to the next song worked up to a point but there were several instances when she wanted to leave. Remembering that Alice thought that she wasn't ill, that this admission was entirely unnecessary and was a general waste of her time and everyone else's, I took her by the hand, and we walked down a long corridor and admired the artwork on the walls.

It made no difference as when we returned, the jiggling of her legs recommenced. She made the same statements and I started to get grumpy.

If we weren't sitting in a hospital admission room, it would have been easier but sitting with someone who is in the throes of psychosis is difficult. There was no way I could have stayed there if it was just the two of us. I needed Shane to be there to support us both. His words of wisdom and his gentle but firm way of dealing with Alice's desire to leave were a relief to me.

I was so grateful when her name was called, I nearly jumped to my feet and wanted to punch the air and yell *BINGO*. I reluctantly refrained. The lovely administration man apologised for the delay and explained that the paperwork was now completed.

We then waited for a porter to walk us to her ward. The process had taken so long that Shane had to leave us to make an appointment at work after he walked with us to her room.

We meandered down the corridors, from the private hospital through to the public hospital and back to where the private and public intermingle with doctors' rooms, outpatient facilities and the mental health wing. We passed by the beautiful prints on the wall, and on the floor there was a vivid carpet that meandered and changed, winding its way to USpace. The porter gave us some information about the ward and how lovely it would be. She also told us that Alice was the third patient that she had walked there this morning. I had seen what it looked like from pictures online, but would it be the same in reality? Would it be better than the PECC unit?

The corridor finally ended at a lift in a relatively new building and we took the lift to the USpace floor. When the doors opened, it was to an entrance filled with sunlight from an enclosed secure courtyard surrounded with glass walls. There was a glass security door where you pushed an intercom button to speak to the receptionist or nurse on duty. They look at you from their secure position inside to see who it is, then ask who you are and buzz you in.

We arrived into the most warm and friendly atmosphere. Greeted at the door with a gentle smile from a kind Irish nurse, who was a few years older than me. She took us on a tour of the facility and talked to Alice directly, not to me, which is the way it should be. I just listened.

My heart no longer felt so heavy.

Our girl still thought all she needed was yoga. As if hearing this thought, the nurse told us there were Pilates, art classes and walks available when she was well enough. There would be group discussions on dealing with the different aspects of mental illness and there was also something for Shane, Harry, and me. A meeting on Friday afternoons for families. The first tiny bit of help that I had heard for us and the only help that we had been offered as a family. These Friday meetings were only being held for the first time and the powers that be were hoping they would be helpful for families and friends, just like us.

The best way to describe Uspace was that was very much like a hostel, *not* like a hospital. There was someone's guitar in the hallway, puzzles on a shelf along with about a hundred books: a mini library filled with Harry Potter, mysteries, romances and young adult novels. A reading room was painted vibrantly and had a couple of large bean bags. There were washing machines and dryers, an outdoor area with tables and chairs if you needed to breathe in fresh air. There was a small kitchen for the catering staff and a dining room that seated twenty in-patients and, finally, just a sliver of one of the best views in Sydney, a view of Sydney Harbour.

The nurse asked Alice if she wanted me with her as they would need to go through her medical history. Alice agreed to let me to stay and we were taken into a small room to be admitted. Alice's vital signs, her blood pressure, pulse, temperature, and medical history were taken. Then she recounted her story to the best of her ability. What she could not remember or stuff that was hazy, I tried to fill in. I had also printed out the history that Jesse has taken from Houssain and the crew in Istanbul.

We knew that on her overseas holiday she smoked marijuana and took the Captogen tablet, the drug we thought at that stage tipped her over the edge into psychosis. I was surprised and shocked to hear Alice say that she had been smoking marijuana since she was sixteen years old. I tried to keep my expression neutral as it wasn't the time to judge, it was the time to heal and move on.

So many questions came to my mind though: how we missed such a thing, how she got it and where she smoked it. At the end of the day, it is something I couldn't change, I had to move forward not backward. Don't get me wrong. I wanted to yell at her, *Are you serious!* I wanted to be angry with her too, but at the same time I was angry at myself and Shane for not knowing.

I felt relieved that the medical staff would get to the issues, to start the healing process of mind, body and soul.

The registered nurse (RN) in charge of the ward came and introduced herself to us. While the admission nurse took Alice to her room, the RN told me that she would find the perfect psychiatrist for Alice's needs. There were a few to choose from but she had a specific one in mind and would workshop her idea with her nursing team when they got Alice's entire history.

As Alice was an adult, they asked her if she wanted to share her medical information with Shane and me, making her fully aware that she didn't need to if she didn't want to. Fortunately for us she allowed us the right to know her medical information, other than the details of her psychiatric appointments. If she wanted us to be privy to what went on in those meetings, she could tell us herself or give permission to the psychiatrist to share with us.

It was clear we had lots of mending of mind and spirits to do, and an enormous amount of investigating to educate us as well. It was time to roll our sleeves up and get down to business. We hoped that the psychiatrist and medical staff would be up for the challenge, that Alice was up for a different kind of adventure and most importantly, she would believe us, rather than the psychotic thoughts that raced through her brain.

We finished the tour and admission process and Alice was taken to her room, right next to the nurses' station. This was so they could observe her, as she needed to be monitored closely. She was the sickest patient in the unit at that time, although she was blissfully unaware of the importance of the position of her room. In those first few days Alice was monitored hourly. The observations were not intrusive, they were visual and verbal checks, and the staff would ask her questions that monitored her mental health and wellbeing.

The bedroom door was beautifully panelled, and the small room had a window seat where the sun left sparkles of light on the fabric. There she could listen to her music or draw. When her mind stopped aching, there was also a television. There was a bedside table for her trinkets, and a little portable clock that I purchased so she could see the time. There was no cord with the clock. She could bring whatever she wanted from home, pillows, blankets, doonas, anything to make her feel more comfortable and settled.

Though time had dragged so slowly during the general admission process that morning, it had flown once we arrived at USpace and soon it would be lunch.

The nurse suggested that it was probably a great time for me to go and let Alice settle into her new environment.

I hugged her and told her Shane would be back in the afternoon on his way home to check in on her.

We walked to the *say goodbye* door. As the nurse released the lock to let me out, I watched Alice turn and slowly walk back down the hallway.

When I pressed the lift button, I hoped that that place would bring the answers to some of our questions. To be honest, at that moment all I wanted was a magic wand and some fairy dust to make it all better and back to what it was before.

I felt the heaviness in my heart and the weight on my shoulders lift just a little. We still needed something to help us through this minefield as a family. We needed tools to deal with her mental ill health and tools to help us withstand the barrage of negative missiles that our girl lobbed at us relentlessly.

Occasionally she would apologise when she could see that she had gone too far. I knew that she didn't mean to be nasty or hurtful. She just couldn't stop the awful vitriol that came out of her mouth. We had no doubt that she loved us but at that time we felt that she didn't like us. The feeling was mutual.

***

Thursday 17 September 2015

In the morning when I visited Alice, the nursing unit manager came out to tell me that she thought she had the perfect psychiatrist for Alice, Dr Leticia Aydos. She would see Alice that afternoon. I could only trust that would happen and couldn't wait to hear what Alice thought of her.

A couple of hours later one of the nurses rang me to say that Dr Leticia had seen Alice and was very optimistic with her progress. She was still a high-risk patient with the nurses continuing their hourly observations, which were just going in to say hello and check on her mental state. At that stage they thought the psychosis would resolve as her clarity was a little better.

Dr Aydos, or Dr Leticia as we would come to call her, started Alice on 200 mg of Epilim, a mood stabiliser, used in conjunction with her antipsychotic drugs. They had started to decrease the antipsychotic drug Olanzapine from 17.5 mg to 15 mg and would gradually get it down to 7.5 mg if possible. One of the nurses explained to me that studies showed that using these two drugs in conjunction could increase the improvement in patients. We were aware that these drugs might not work for Alice. It was going to be a matter of trial, error, an abundance of patience and I think a sprinkle of good luck thrown in for good measure.

At this facility, as was the case at the PECC unit, you couldn't have plastic bags, scissors, nail scissors, nail clippers of any kind or anything sharp. She could have her phone, which was her lifeline to Houssain. He was her constant calm and the one person who listened to her ramblings and her moments of sanity, but sadly he was so very far away.

Dr Leticia explained drug-induced psychosis to us. She said that you could have twenty people in a room that all took the same drug, even the same dosage, but out of all those people, one person in that room might react differently and that person, this time, was Alice.

I send off a quick text to Houssain, who was sometimes more in the loop than we were, as Alice kept him up to date with all that was going on, including her delusions. He continued to be so patient and calm with Alice, listening to her and talking with her until she settled.

***

It was hard for us to hear of the unrest in Turkey that was attributed to the Syrian refugees who had arrived needing asylum from their war-ravaged country. We listened to the horrific stories of the men, women and children escaping on the boats to Greece, and some drowning as the result of overcrowding when boats tragically sank. These people were so desperate to escape war and unimaginable happenings and horrors in their home country, to start a new life, that they attempted to get to any country that would have them, risking their safety. Their desperation was real and horrifying for us to watch even from afar. We could only imagine what it had been like for our Syrian crew.

***

Alice's days were filled with nothingness. Her sadness and frustration at not being able to use her brain as it hurt too much was palpable. Her concentration span was still short. Doing simple things that we take for granted like reading a magazine or writing in her much-loved journal or doing a puzzle were at that stage an impossibility.

All she had to entertain herself were her eyes, her music, Houssain and the voices in her head.

Her annoyance was obvious and understandable.

On occasion Alice would say that she was a burden and we told her that wasn't true. We wanted her to get better, but we just didn't know when that would be. One of the positives about being in hospital was that there was always one of the wonderful nurses around to share our concerns with. They would go sit and speak with her about what she was feeling and tell her she was not alone.

A week into her stay, she said we were visiting too much. She was right. I was going in the morning or in the afternoon if I was working and Shane would go after work. The truth was that it made me feel less guilty if I went to see her. I felt like we had had her locked up and I *had* to visit her. I said we could call her every morning, and she could let us know if she was up for a visit that day.

***

Mid-September 2015

Alice

When I was in the hospital, I still felt like I was being tested. A delusion had stuck with me from being in the Bull: that I had to survive this for the sake of all lives taken through suicide. I was being tested mostly through technology. I remember scrolling through my Spotify playlist and feeling like I was being observed by aliens who wanted to harvest my soul and predict the moves I was making, down to even the order of songs I would play. Recurring numbers remained a problem. One night while I was trying to take a selfie to send to Houssain, the Egyptian ankh (key of life symbol) appeared falling over my head, like a shower of rain. Obviously, this was a hallucination, but it felt so real. I had promised to talk to a nurse every time something wigged me out. So, I would go to the nurse and she would assure me I was in a safe place, and I was then able to return to my room. Though what I really wanted to do was sleep on the couch in the corridor.

The next day, I thought I heard some girls call me a foetus because of my rough mental state. I tried having a conversation with them as I thought they would understand the alien delusion, but clearly their comprehension of the matter was zero, so I learnt then that it was a restricted topic and not everyone was on the same wavelength as me.

Sarah

Alice saw her psychiatrist once a day during the week, and her diagnosis remained the same, that Alice had suffered from a drug-induced psychosis due to the drug Captagon. Dr Leticia could not rule out signs of bipolar disorder. She told us that it could take years before a definitive diagnosis was made. In the meantime, Shane and I continued googling and reading any and all information that we could get our hands on.

CHAPTER 22

Out for lunch

Wednesday 23 September 2015

Sarah

I arrived one glorious sun filled morning, and the nurses suggested that Alice could go out on leave for a couple of hours. So why not go out for lunch. I was excited that Alice could do something different with her day and that I would be involved.

I asked her what she wanted like to do, forgetting that her decision-making capability was zero. Thinking I was doing the right thing, I suggested lunch at Kings Cross. A gentle walk of around ten minutes and then to a café. No big deal.

HUGE mistake.

I realised this as soon as we got twenty metres out of the front entrance of the hospital, when we stopped at a set of traffic lights.

A car horn blared loudly behind us. A couple were having an argument, and someone jostled past us as we crossed the road. Alice was holding my hand nervously. Her eyes were darting from one noise to the next. Instead of re-evaluating, I decided to press on. Dragging Alice with me, with no thought or regard to how overwhelming it must have been for her.

Situation and noise overload.

There was way too much going on.

Too much hustle.

Too much bustle.

And too many people.

Way, way too many people.

Oddly, I was trying to make it a positive experience and I pushed on, determined to have lunch with my girl. Not realising the stress and anxiety I was putting her under, and me too for that matter. I hadn't yet realised that this was our new normal: to expect the unexpected and change the game plan when necessary, always moving forwards and not backwards. I would come to learn that it's okay to move sideways, lick our wounds and retreat, but had not twigged to this on that day.

We stopped at a burger place a slow ten-minute walk from the hospital and ordered our meals. By that stage Alice was agitated and ready to leave and yet we had only just arrived. I was at a loss. She got up to go once, and I took her hand and asked her to stay. I had visions of when we were in Istanbul at the restaurant. I realised then how unprepared I was.

It was loud. The sounds reverberated against the walls and tiled floors. The clang of the plates, a coffee machine pumping out cappuccinos and to top it off we were sitting at a long, shared table. Ten different groups of people all talked at once, and then there was the music coming out of the ceiling somewhere.

I held her hand, thankful she had her headphones on to block everything out. I couldn't ask her to take them off, so I texted Shane, explaining in detail the unfolding disaster.

All I could think about was what a fool I was. I needed it to work out in order to feel like progress had been made, so when things weren't going to plan, I wasn't flexible enough to change course.

My big mistake was I had not asked for suggestions from the nurses, and I had taken Alice out for her first outing by myself.

A rookie error on my part.

Lunch tasted like cardboard. The relief we both felt just leaving the burger place was immediate. Surprisingly, we both couldn't wait to get back to USpace.

A hard lesson was learned: always prepare ahead of time and without a doubt have a plan B and C up your sleeve.

Alice went into her room, and I got us both a cup of tea and spoke with one of the nurses about our awful hour on day leave.

The day RN, of course, said it had been a bad move and then suggested the beach, or the park, and there was this peaceful little courtyard at the art school just around the corner. That would have been perfect. And helpful to know before I took her out. It really had been one of those throw your arms in the air and raise your eyes to the sky moments, while slapping my palm against my forehead.

Note to self: if in doubt, ask.

Those people were there to help.

***

Saturday 26 September 2015

Alice got another leave pass for a few hours, so we brought her home. Minnie the dog greeted her at the door like she had been gone forever and stayed by her side the entire time. We loved that she was home. Life for a few hours returned to normal as we sat down to lunch outside. We talked, listened to the neighbourhood dogs barking and cooked on the BBQ which created the occasional whoosh of smoke in our faces. We all laughed at Shane, getting great joy in telling him he should have at least moved the BBQ further away from the table. Meanwhile Minnie waited patiently for a tasty morsel to fall her way.

Life in that moment, on the surface, appeared so very normal.

We FaceTimed Jesse and Ella in Melbourne and while we were talking Alice said that day reminded her of when they were in Krka National Park in Croatia. They all collaborated to tell us the Krka National Park story, as Al could not tell the whole story without help. In that moment life seemed so normal and I felt at peace.

CHAPTER 23

Flashback: Krka National Park

24 June 2015, Krka, Croatia

Alice, Jesse and Ella

In Croatia, our first stop was Krka National Park, where we went to see the most breathtaking, spectacular waterfalls. We spent the day lazing in the water and on the rocks. Four Australians at a water feature meant four above-average swimmers. We thought the line of buoys about thirty metres away from the falls was just a guide to where the water was shallow. So, naturally, we swam the gap to sit under the falling water.

The time that we sat in the falls was bliss. That special white noise of water, the opalescent blue of it and all of this in the middle of a dense, green rainforest. Then a whistle blew. And again. And again. We realised a man in khakis was yelling and gesturing to us.

The line of buoys was a 'do not cross' type of situation … The poor man had no idea what reaction he had just set off though. The whistling alerted most people at the waterfall to the fact that there was a group of four sitting under the falls. The most picturesque place in an already picturesque place! Almost everyone with a GoPro started their own dash to the falls, while we rode the current back to the safe side of the buoys.

The whistling man kept whistling. But the flood had started, people from all along the one hundred metres of rope ducked under and swam over to try to find their own spot of bliss. The whistling man didn't know what to do. He dove in the water with all his clothes still on and demanded everyone return.

Finally, having everyone back on the right side of the rope, he took his shirt off and stood on a shallow rock. He was the whistling guardian of the falls. We had started a mob and he had to clean up the mess. We felt bad, but at the same time the whole situation was hilarious and nobody got hurt. The law of unintended consequences can sometimes throw up chaos. Hopefully the whistler won employee of the month for his hard work and wet clothes!!!

CHAPTER 24

A gift

Saturday 26 September 2015

Sarah

When Alice, Jess and Ella told us the story about Krka, it was the most Alice had spoken in weeks. What a beautiful and funny story to be able to share with us, and how wonderful that her brother was able to share that moment with her too. It was a positive flash of hope in a hard week.

When it came to returning to the unit, Alice wanted to know why she couldn't stay at home. She continued to be unable to see that she was ill. Diplomacy was needed and I outsourced that to Shane. I was all done being diplomatic. As much as I wanted to get her to go back, I couldn't drag her there and my patience had been exhausted. Shane was matter of fact and all business. We both took her back and Minnie the dog would come for the drive and stay in the car while Shane walked Alice back to Uspace and signed her in.

If we thought the dark tentacles were loosening, we needed to think again.

***

Monday 28 September 2015

The next week followed in much the same routine: same, same but different. On Monday, she was again allowed out for a few hours leave. Over the phone Alice and I discussed what she wanted to do and agreed that our last outing to Kings Cross was an unmitigated disaster.

That day we would go for a walk around Centennial Park, a huge park in Sydney's eastern suburbs. I packed a bag with a thermos of tea, took two mugs, some biscuits and tucked a rug under my arm.

We found a beautiful spot on the grass where we could watch the ducks around the lake and some delightful young children trying to feed them. We listened to the birds squawking, dogs barking in the distance, kids squealing and laughing and heard the steady clip clop of a couple of horses out for an afternoon trot. The weather was overcast and cool but the gentle breeze on our faces was healing. It was lovely to have some time out in the fresh air – that is until the heavens opened up and the rain arrived. So, with both of us yelling, grabbing the thermos, rug, and each other's hands, we made a mad but invigorating dash to the car about a kilometre away. Breathless and laughing, we arrived soaked but with smiles splattered all over our faces and there was huge love in my heart. It was the first time in a month that I had heard Alice laugh. I would keep it locked in my memory for the next little while, until another precious moment could be added to it.

Alice spent another week in the hospital. Dr Leticia was still unsure what her final diagnosis was or what conclusion to draw from what had happened. She was positive with the progress Al had made. She reminded us that it was a marathon, not a sprint. The jury was seemingly out regarding psychosis on its own. Drug-induced psychosis or bipolar in conjunction with psychosis looked most likely. That appeared to be the 'thing' with mental health, a diagnosis takes time and patience and of that we had plenty.

At this time, I couldn't say what Alice thought of her psychiatrist. I did know that Shane and I had an enormous amount of respect and admiration for her. Dr Leticia had met us and discussed all the pros and cons of psychosis, drug-induced psychosis and bipolar as diagnoses. She talked with us, not at us, and was interested in what we had to say, which, to be honest, was not much at that stage. She wanted to be informed if we thought anything had changed regarding Alice, or if we thought she as a doctor could do something better.

CHAPTER 25

Alice comes home

Friday 2 October 2015

Sarah

After seventeen days of intensive psychiatric treatment, medical procedures and examinations to rule out any other diagnosis, and scans done of her brain, Alice was discharged from USpace.

When I collected her, we gave the nurses a big box of Krispy Kreme doughnuts. We thanked them for all their care and support and to not take it personally, but we hoped to never return.

It was a wonderful day.

There is no quick fix with mental illness. Alice still heard voices. Her thoughts were scattered and her frustration high and her anger obvious. She was still very ill but able to be released into our care.

Alice would continue to see Dr Leticia twice a week and a

psychologist, Ms J, once a week. Ms J was from the First Episode of Psychosis program at the public hospital where Alice was first admitted and treated. This treatment was free and an initiative from the Australian Government. It was a godsend. My entire wage went to paying the psychiatrist's fees. There is no way we would have been able to afford psychology payments as well.

Ms J was a wonderful psychologist who I felt we were lucky to have been assigned. She would come to our home, or meet Alice in a coffee shop, or wherever Alice would like to meet. When she came to our home, they would sit outside for an hour while she worked her magic with our girl, simply by listening to her.

Twice a week I drove Alice to see Dr Leticia at her rooms at St Vincent's Hospital. I'd sit in the waiting room and read until Alice came out. In the following weeks, Dr Leticia was hopeful that Alice would be able to start driving herself to the appointments. When that could happen, we would know that the fog was lifting and maybe the tentacles were slowly losing their grip around her.

Small steps, going forward.

***

October 2015

Alice

When I was discharged from hospital, I was still in the grip of psychosis but well enough not to need the full-time supervision or care of a hospital setting, and for that I was appreciative.

A month after I got out, an uncomfortable experience occurred when I decided to go to a friend's house. I had been given the green light to drive, which gave me added freedom, so I picked up one of my friends and we drove to Coogee for a party, about a forty-five-minute drive from my house.

When we were there, I felt overwhelmed by all the people. I believed that people could hear my thoughts and that there were terrorists listening in. I was sure my friend was in danger of being targeted by the terrorists, being mistaken for me, just for being in the same car.

I had no headphones so there was no music in my ears to divert my thoughts.

My friend was oblivious and I was terrified that the bad guys were coming.

I spent the first thirty minutes wandering the periphery of the party, looking for threats. Then an hour sitting in a corner with an exuberant bunch of people, trying to be as invisible as possible. Hiding in plain sight, all the while trying to build up the courage to leave.

Finally, after a few hours, I found my friend and told her I was going and asked if she'd like a lift home, glad she did as I thought she was in danger.

My delusions did not end when we left.

On the drive home, I believed that all the number plates of cars were spelling out secret codes and messages for me.

I assumed that I was able to hide what was going on around me as my friend appeared to be oblivious to the crisis that she was sitting next to. She did not ask if I was okay or question any of my actions.

I felt so awkward, monitoring my own movements and the movements of those around me. In hindsight, it was like I was trying to conceal the illness or that the illness was trying not to be spotted by those around me. It was in fact consuming my social life.

I observed myself observing how other people observed me and I became paranoid and self-conscious. Though I was more self-aware than ever, the healing process had been a vague nightmare. Yet I wish I could have remembered more of the secret delusions I held wrapped away in my feeble mind. Sometimes I doubted myself and thought I could still look at things and see so much meaning.

Sarah

The Olanzapine continued to make Alice very sleepy. Fortunately, her psychiatrist listened to what Al had to say and changed her medication to another antipsychotic drug called Abilify that was taken in the morning. I was relieved that someone heard what Alice said and acted upon it. We needed to wait a few weeks to see the difference, if any, that the new drug made.

Shane works at a company called TOGA. They were absolutely amazing. They offered to help in any way they could and allowed him to work from home when he deemed it necessary. It was a stress reliever for us both. They were also supportive, asking him how we all were coping.

During this first month that Alice was home from the hospital, one of us wanted to be with her. Shane worked from home a few days a week, so I could go back to work. I dropped down to working two, ten-hour days a week. It was a relief for me to return to my usual routine. Fortunately, working in healthcare had its advantages. It made it so easy to tell my intimate group of five work colleagues (the ones that sent the flowers), a surgeon, anaesthetist, scrub nurse, scout nurse and anaesthetic nurse in my theatre, what was going on. At that time, they were the only people outside my family that knew exactly what was happening. They were, in fact, under a vow of silence, to not speak with any of our colleagues as to what was happening in my home life. So worried was I about the stigma of mental health.

I was glad to be there but anxious to get back home too.

Surprisingly, it was the little things that I have found the hardest. Top of the list was that it was unbelievably hard to keep a smile on my face and have a positive attitude a hundred percent of the time at home. I liken it to hosting a party or your wedding day. By the end of the night, you have had a great time, but your cheeks are aching from smiling, laughing, chatting, making sure everyone is having a good time. I was doing that all day, every day.

I'd get my mask in place as I made my way home from work. When I got home, I'd take a deep breath, open the front door and see what awaited me there.

One afternoon on our walk, Alice opened up to me about something that happened at the beginning of 2015. She said she was at a party and heard voices in her head. She felt scared but thought she had had too much to drink and convinced herself her head was ok. It happened again a few weeks before she left for overseas but she put it down to the stress of her final exams. It didn't happen again before she left so she said nothing. Why did Alice say *nothing?* She was scared if she voiced her concerns to us, that she wouldn't be able to go on her well-deserved holiday. So, she remained silent.

The confusion, fear and angst she must have grappled with, not to say anything, was horrifying to now know.

We stopped walking and I hugged her.

She told me she had spoken with Dr Leticia about it.

We moved forward.

On another day Alice and I went for a walk on a path that weaves its way around some water. We had one of those great chats that parents love. I didn't talk, I just listened. I had found out that Alice had trod a rough and rocky path in her teenage years and we had no inkling. This was when Alice opened up about why she stopped swimming as a teenager and the bullying that had occurred.

I also didn't listen when she wanted to switch schools in her teens. In my mind, as a mother, I could not see what was wrong with her current school. I didn't *hear* her and her heartfelt words.

Could we have made those years any different for her?

I am unsure, but we could have made them easier for her if we had *really* heard her.

Listening to our children and hearing what they are truly saying is probably one of the greatest things that we can do for them.

We cannot live on should have, would have, or could have, but we can choose to be honest, attentive and positive. To grow and move forward to not be afraid to laugh, to cry, to be angry and to be sad. Most importantly to question when the need arises.

As the season moved towards summer, psychosis still sat at our table. The tentacles were wrapped firmly around her. Alice would talk about learning Arabic, making plans to get Houssain to Australia. Then thirty minutes later she'd tell me that she was going to tell Houssain not to message her anymore. We had come to know that this was all part of her illness, we were ready for these changes of mood and mind. We were learning to live with them, like an unwelcome flatmate that paid no rent. Tolerated but not welcomed.

She was still getting angry. There were brief bursts of anger, like a rant for a minute or so, but at times this anger would go on for an hour. When this happened there was nowhere for me to go. Houssain was amazing. I am sure there must have been many times when he questioned his relationship with Alice and what his role in her life was and what it should be, but at that time he was her friend, her ally, and her rock.

***

November 2015

Sarah

By November we started leaving Alice alone at home during the day while we were at work. Some days I dreaded leaving her, although talk of suicide had only been mentioned by her just that once. We did know she battled with the state of her mind every minute of every day. There were times when Shane or I would go to work and one of us would return home several hours later, due to the state of her mental health not being positive or receiving a text from her that concerned us.

Alice knew that her mind was still a jigsaw and bits of the puzzle were not slotting into the correct spots. It had her frustrated at not being 'normal', wanting her mind to be healthy but also knowing that it would take time, and that time was taking too long. Even after a few months Alice was still unable to do 'stuff', like read a book, watch a simple television show from start to finish or draw in the adult colouring-in books, as concentrating continued to exhaust her brain.

What were we to do?

What was she to do?

We told her that having mental ill health did not define who she was. She needed patience, resilience and above all to trust in us. With psychotic thoughts and voices still racing through her mind, she needed an enormous amount of mental strength to hear and believe what we were saying to hear. Some days she heard us, some days … she did not.

We had to keep chipping away and hold on to the hope that we clutched valiantly in our hands and in our hearts.

We were all in this fight together, Alice, Shane, Harry, me and from afar, Jesse and Ella.

Once a day we walked. Fortunately, down the end of our street is a beautiful bush walk that I hadn't known about. Alice took me there one day, it runs parallel to the water, so it was refreshingly beautiful. The trees between the bay and the dirt path gave us little glimpses of the water. We would take Minnie the dog with us. As the weeks went by, Alice would go for a walk by herself, taking Minnie with her. Minnie was my safety net, so Alice was never alone.

We would talk and agree on a list of things for her to achieve the next day. Very simple things so as not to overtax her mind. Colouring in her books, getting out of her pyjamas, stacking the dishwasher after a meal, going for a walk, sitting outside in the sun, and lastly seeing if she could read one page from a book. Most of the time it was only one thing that got done on any given day, but we counted that as an achievement.

Dr Leticia impressed on us how well Alice was doing and reminded us that she had been compliant with taking her medication, went to her appointments three times a week, and was doing everything within her ability to fight this battle with all the strength she could at that moment.

We just wanted her back.

We wanted her in a place where she felt safe, worthwhile, loved, and important.

We had been told by Dr Leticia to take things very slowly and not to expect much. The extent of her brain recovery, how functioning she would become, and her mental health recovery was an unknown to us all.

So, we became her everything in those first months.

We were her parents, her family, her friends, her confidants, her antagonists, her chains, but mostly we were the source of unconditional love. As frustratingly slow as her healing was, ultimately, I truly believe we were her strength when she could not find it in herself.

What we needed to remember was that we were only ten weeks post-psychosis. The recovery that Alice had made was amazing and awe-inspiring.

Outwardly to the world, the people that we walked past in the streets, not one person would have had any idea that the girl walking beside me, had been in the fight of her life and in our eyes, she was WINNING.

CHAPTER 26

Friends

Sarah

One of the things that saddened me was the behaviour of some of Alice's friends.

The friends that disappeared. What could have been done to keep them around? I suspect nothing. Fair-weather friends will always be just that.

What it meant though was potential loneliness and sadness for our girl.

A few of the friends that we had contacted while we were at Istanbul Airport visited her in hospital and after her discharge came over to our house a few times, but then they became suddenly silent. I can only assume that it was too hard and perhaps too confronting for them to deal with this stranger that Alice had become to them.

As a mother I wanted to speak to them and ask where they were. Why they were not supporting my girl. Their friendship was over ten years in the making so I presumed the bonds were strong. Sadly, they were not.

A few other friends would ask her to lunch, coffee or to the beach, not regularly but at least they asked her out. Ultimately getting her out of the house. For that, I am grateful.

The handful of special people that have supported Alice has been a surprise and these wonderful humans fill our hearts with joy and a special place in in our hearts is just for them.

Her foremost constant friend was a young lady by the name of Lozza, that Alice has been friends with since they met in first grade. They went to different schools from the age of thirteen but kept in contact throughout. Lozza and her wonderful family have passed no judgement on Alice, not once. She was so happy to see and hear from Alice and she is worth a million smiles and hugs from me.

Her other friends Sam and JD, like Lozza, have been honest and true to Alice, supporting her when she was down and being there for her on the good days as well as the bad.

They would come and see her, they would ask her to gatherings, parties or simply just to hang out. Their names make me smile every time I hear them, and they will forever be welcome in our home.

Abbey, who Alice had met in Istanbul, came to see her. She lives a few hours away and that was no mean feat. She was sad to see Alice like she was. Lena, a lovely friend that had moved to Germany was concerned and worried but felt helpless to do anything. She would text Alice and then she would text me asking how exactly

Alice was going. As did Francesca, an Italian girl that Alice had met and stayed with in Milan a few years previously.

What they did was show they cared. Oh, how I wished they lived in Sydney!

Crowds and noise still caused her anxiety, so going out in groups, to pubs or parties had to wait. She had learnt to get there on time but to leave early before the noise started. There was also the added concern from me about drugs being present. Even the thought of her being around people who took drugs was enough to give me a migraine.

Alice and I had an open discussion regarding drugs, alcohol, and friends.

I voiced my concern to her.

Are there drugs around?

If there are, what do you do?

What coping strategies will you use?

I was concerned with the answers she would give me, but we had ditched the burying of our heads in the sand months ago. Honesty was our best and only policy.

She answered yes to being in all of these situations. The hard answers to my questions were that these were people that she liked. They knew her situation, that if she took drugs that the very real result could be that she could have another drug-induced psychosis. She said she had been offered marijuana but said no. She said I needed to let her go and trust in her ability to say *no*.

So that is what we did, trust.

I followed that discussion with what I felt was a heartfelt plea.

"I need to say this to you.

"I am terrified that if you take drugs, that we will not get you back again. I feel incredibly blessed that we got you back this time but if it were to happen again, we do not know what the result would be and, Alice, I do not know if I can go through that again."

We hugged and Al said she had no desire for this to happen again either.

Ultimately it is Alice who makes her decisions, not us. She is in control of her destiny, and no matter what we say or do, it is her choice.

I also had the embarrassing 'mum' talk with two of her friends, Sam and JD, about drugs and Alice not going together. I am not sure whether they gave me lip service just to appease me. Although they were as concerned with her welfare as we were.

CHAPTER 27

Turning point

January 2016

Sarah

January brought hot weather and a beach holiday up the north coast at a place called Boomerang Beach, a three-hour drive from our home in Sydney.

It's a place that embodies peace and tranquillity. With the sun shining, great surf, sand and beautiful bush walks, we'd recharge our batteries.

One day on our walk we stopped at the local shops and the owner of the local café was lamenting that he had a delivery of equipment but that the instructions were in Italian.

At that time, Alice was suffering greatly from the voices, depression, low self-esteem and a lack of confidence. We couldn't do much to rouse her from its depths. Try as we may, we could not loosen the tentacles that held her so tightly.

Unaware of how Alice was feeling, this random shop owner inadvertently did something none of us had thought to do to increases her confidence. He actually said, "Does anyone here speak Italian?" Alice speaks Italian fluently.

She offered to translate it for him but told him she'd look at it that night and be back the next morning with her translation.

He was surprised and grateful to her and gave her free coffee for the rest of our vacation.

To us, it was a special moment in her brain recovery, perhaps the first real change that we had seen. This was the first time that someone had come to Alice requiring HER assistance. It made her feel important, needed and valued. We were so proud, especially knowing the hours of mental energy that she put into translating the document.

It also showed us how important it is to feel needed and wanted, to be valued in any situation. We had forgotten this in all our dealings. We kept saying Alice was in control of her destiny and it really was true. But we needed to step back and keep this in the forefront of our minds and let her be her, to start to be her own person again.

While we were away, Alice decided that she wanted to teach English as a second language. She did a lot of investigating and research on Google and I was able to contact an old school friend, Kate, who taught English in Italy and asked what course she thought was the best to do.

Alice did more research on the CELTA (Certificate in Teaching English to Adults), and then sent in an application. Much to her surprise, while we were still in Boomerang Beach, she got a response and had an interview lined up several days after our return.

CHAPTER 28

Study

February 2016

Sarah

On the day of Alice's CELTA interview, she became extremely anxious. It was a gently, gently approach that got her out the door. She drove to the station, got on the train and went for her interview BY HERSELF. Another small step but a MAJOR life-changing moment for Alice.

A week later, she was accepted into the course, to commence in ten days, full-time for four weeks.

It became glaringly obvious after the first day of lectures that getting through the next nineteen days, roughly one hundred and fifty-two hours, would be a nightmare. If it was bad for Alice, that meant that it was bad for us too.

Back-to-back classes, the only relief being a scheduled break for lunch, was going to be a God Almighty struggle for her. The classes were full-on. Alice's mind had not been switched on for six months and had sustained a great mental trauma. Suddenly, it was full steam ahead.

We had a discussion after the second day about whether it was worth continuing.

The stress and anxiety Alice felt was alarming.

I lamented the fact that the course could not be done part-time and Alice said, "Oh, but you can, Mum, I just thought it would be better to get it over and done with."

A part-time course would have been the better option, but we saw it for what it was, Alice standing on her own feet, making decisions.

I sent an urgent text to Dr Leticia, not because of her decision-making, but in just two short days her anxiety and depression had her at an all-time low. We had not seen her like that in months and it was extremely concerning.

Fortunately, Alice had an appointment after her classes with Dr Leticia that afternoon and they would workshop the best scenario for moving forward.

The next day, three days after commencing her full-time course, she trudged off to class. The dark tentacles were firmly around her shoulders and defeat was in her every step. But she had a question, *'Can I defer and change to part-time?'*

The answer was yes and yes, but a request for approval needed to be sent to head office in Cambridge in the United Kingdom.

***

March 2016

We discussed exactly what Alice wanted to do. The logical answer was to stop and restart the course later and do it part-time. But it was Alice who needed to make the decision, not us. We discussed the three previous days, and how she felt. We asked if she was to measure the stress and anxiety out of ten, what would it be? The course was not going to get any easier. In fact, with exams to come, it was only going to become harder. With much heartache, she decided it would be best to defer. The decision came with mixed emotions as she felt like a failure, a loser and a fool all rolled into one.

Yet, even with Alice feeling those emotions, we as parents felt so much pride in what she had achieved. To us, she had not failed. To us, she truly had taken a giant leap forward in her mental and emotional recovery. We kept telling her that we could not be prouder. Alice, of course, could not understand this, she could only see the negative. The tentacles were forming a cloak over her and the remaining voices in her head encouraged them.

The next day, she went off to class to inform the course educator that she would be deferring and would re-enrol in the next part-time course in late May. This decision gave Alice something positive and worthwhile to look forward to.

For the last five months, Alice had been tracking all of her Syrian friends that she had met in Turkey. One by one, most of them had left on the dangerous, shonky boats that fled Turkish waters in the deepest, darkest of night. Boatloads of desperate and displaced Syrians wanting to find better lives for themselves and their families.

Every time one of her friends made the crossing from Turkey to Greece, Alice would anxiously await the news that they had arrived safely.

The trip was made even scarier due to the condition of the boats, frequently breaking apart, taking on water and sinking, with not a life jacket in sight.

This crossing was made by nearly one million Syrian refugees in 2015 and 2016. Heartbreakingly, the majority of the refugees could not swim. They were leaving Turkey to find a better life, or simply a safe life for themselves, and hopefully reunite with family and friends.

All while the rest of the world watched on with most nations doing nothing.

The night finally came when it was Houssain's turn. He had decided that there was nothing left in Istanbul for him. Most of his friends had left, his family were already elsewhere in Europe, and he wanted to find them and see them again. There was talk of the so-called borders shutting down. So, there was an urgency to his leaving. He needed to get out in the next week or he would be stuck in Turkey for the foreseeable future.

Alice waited anxiously by her phone, keeping us updated on any news. In this case, no news was definitely not good, and until he arrived safely, we would worry.

We will never know the terror that he faced that night, to get on the boat or the ordeal he had suffered in Syria years before. We do know that this man deserved the freedom of the world and the right to be wherever he chose.

He travelled on one of the last refugee boats out of Turkey and made it to Greece. All his possessions from his thirty years wrapped in one tiny backpack. Family documents rolled and wrapped in plastic, his only precious cargo.

The rest of his possessions had been given away to friends that had stayed behind in Istanbul.

It was with a happy heart that Alice was able to tell us one morning that the trip had been a success. Houssain was now firmly on dry land in Greece.

In Greece, he visited the department of immigration every day for months to get a passport. He would stand in horrendous queues for hours each day, only to be told, no, come back tomorrow. It seemed futile as he was getting nowhere.

Literally on the day he was going to give up, luck fell on his side when he met a retired Greek legal aid officer who happened to stand behind him in the queue. They talked and he asked Houssain what his story was. This chance meeting ended up being the miracle that Houssain needed and this wonderful man assisted with him to get a passport to leave Greece.

It was then off to Berlin for Houssain, where he would live with friends until he could find his feet and then reunite with his family.

**

May 2016

Psychotic thoughts and voices still filled Alice's mind, but the antipsychotic medication was weaving its magic and kept Alice stable enough to stay out of hospital and at home. The voices had decreased to one or two and for this we were all grateful. We waited in anticipation for the day when they would all be banished, taking the tentacles with them when they went.

The May CELTA course commencement day arrived and off she went, nervous and excited.

I was so proud.

She met a wonderful English girl, Lorna, who was doing the course and they became fast friends.

Standing up in front of twenty of your peers and teacher is enough to make anyone nervous. Let alone anyone suffering the ravages of mental ill health. Alice had told no one other than Lorna about the road she had travelled to get there. So, the support and encouragement that Lorna gave Alice was priceless.

Make no mistake, Alice got through the course by herself, with her determination and bravery and by facing her fears head on. I do need to note that every day of the course was a battle. I would receive several texts each day that required a positive response of love and encouragement that she could do it. At this time her appointments with Dr Leticia increased to three a week. Financially crippling but worth every cent and extra shifts that I had to work.

***

June 2016

The course finished with Alice passing every aspect of it.

A few weeks later she went for a casual job teaching English as a second language at a college in town. A day later she was informed that she had a job starting the next week if she wanted it. Yes, she did. Three days a week was perfect for her and she commuted into town to educate and teach international students. She loved it and she was earning money for future adventures.

There were so many positives flying through the door, yet we still asked her how she was going every day. There must have been a way we could get around that without asking the same question each day so we didn't drive her to irritation!

I suggested we have a colour-coded bracelet system on the go, where she could put one on each morning to communicate how she was to us without having to verbalise it.

Red for high alert.

Blue for anxiety/depression/voices.

Orange for ok.

Green for calm. s

This was met with ambivalence, so I didn't do anything about it, but in hindsight I think it was a brilliant idea as all we would have to do would be to have a look at her wrist to see how she was rather than constantly asking her.

CHAPTER 29

Houssain

18 September 2016

Sarah

Alice decided that she wanted to see Houssain again. She wanted to see him when she wasn't in the depths of psychosis. To thank him and enjoy time away from home without parental constraints around her. They both wanted to see if a romance, albeit long distance, was worth even thinking about.

She had saved up enough money to get her to Germany and live frugally for three weeks.

She was excited.

I was filled with anxiety.

We made a deal that she would contact us every day and we would do a mental health check to ease my concerns. She would also check in with Dr Leticia.

So nearly a year to the day after she left Istanbul to return home to Sydney in 2015, in September 2016 – armed with her antipsychotic medication, headphones and backpack – she flew to Berlin to spend three weeks with Houssain.

I texted him and he told me he would take great care of her. He was under no illusion about what she had been through. He had been privy to Alice in her darkest places. Now he could hopefully see her in a place of light and happiness.

They were renewing their friendship that had been cut short, robbing them of the chance to see where it might be heading.

Alice was still different to the girl Houssain had first met and loved, but he was so caring, loving and respectful with her that it was hard for us to not love him too.

***

October 2016

On her return, Alice started a permanent job teaching English as a second language in the city, doing a four-day week. There she met a wonderful group of teachers, and with one in particular, called Nicole, she soon became firm friends. Her students loved her and she seemed to have found a small niche in the world for herself.

Some days were good, and some were not. We reminded ourselves: *slow and steady will win this race.*

CHAPTER 30

Saviours

Sarah

I cannot tell you how much we love Houssain and the Syrian crew over in Istanbul. What I need to make clear is that they did not give Alice the Captogon tablet. In fact, when they found out who had given it to her, they stopped all contact with the person.

Ultimately Alice was the one who put the pill in her mouth. She is one hundred percent responsible.

Captagon is was what tipped Alice over the edge into psychosis, but the signs were there already that her mental health was on the precipice. We didn't recognise the signs or see them before she left on her travels and Alice was too scared to go into depth of what they meant.

It now appears to us (good old hindsight) that it was just a matter of time before a psychosis or mental impairment of some sort was going to occur. Remember the conversation Alice had with me on one of our walks about hearing voices before she went overseas?

We will be forever grateful that it happened where and when it did (although Houssain and his friends may wish that it had happened elsewhere!)

If Houssain had not been with her the week leading up to the escalation of her delusional behaviour …

If he hadn't been with her when she tried and go wandering in the middle of night …

If he had not stopped her on the day we flew in from Australia and she had made it into the taxi thinking that she was being chased …

What could have happened to her?

Where would she have asked to be taken to?

Or where would the driver have taken her?

Yes, I have thought through all of these scenarios.

An Aussie girl unwell and lost in a foreign country would no doubt have immediately fallen into the less savoury aspects of life.

She would not have lasted long.

Houssain and our Syrian musketeers will forever have a bed ready in our home if and whenever they visit Australia. I think Houssain would probably be embarrassed to know how much he really is a part of our family and the esteem we hold him in.

Houssain and Alice had a wonderful relationship but sadly it was not to last the tyranny of distance. They have remained friends to this day and I am fortunate to include Houssain as one of mine too.

From *Dear Psychosis,*

I have welcomed the light amidst the darkness.

I have found strength through the anger.

I have embraced the sadness.

I have shouted my grief to the heavens.

I have wiped the tears away.

I will speak.

CHAPTER 31

The future

2017 and 2018

Sarah

Under the guidance of Dr Leticia, Alice slowly came off her anti-anxiety medication in 2017 and in early 2018 she came off her antipsychotic drug Abilify.

In September of 2018, Alice had her second case of psychosis that resulted in a stay in hospital (USpace) where she was then diagnosed with bipolar affective disorder. This is now controlled by Lithium. Oddly, it is a drug that works and we don't know how, only that it does. She is taking this drug in conjunction with Abilify, the antipsychotic medication she was on previously.

Interesting fact for you. In Australia our population is just over twenty-five million people. One percent of the population have bipolar. That's one person in a room of one hundred people!

Alice still sees her fabulous psychiatrist, Dr Leticia Aydos, weekly but no longer sees Ms J her psychologist.

There seems to be a huge misconception that if you have a mental illness that you cannot hold down a job. I have been asked countless times by well-meaning friends if Alice had a job. The answer is the same every time.

Yes, she has been teaching English for the last four years. I still get irritated that this is continually asked.

Yes, she has always taken her medication. In fact, has always been compliant in taking it, even when she was in the throes of psychosis in hospital and that first year of her mental health journey.

I believe that as a family unit we made a great team and certainly have had a huge impact on Alice's health. Ultimately, she is in control of her life and her destiny and knows most of the signs and triggers that she needs to watch for.

We still take one day at a time. There are days where I will need to push her out of bed. Times when the verbal grenades come back. Times when the tentacles of mental ill health hold her hostage. What we have chosen to do is celebrate the good days.

***

October and November 2019

Alice

In late 2019 I travelled to Europe alone for two months. I took my medication with me and was fortunate enough to be able to skype with Dr Leticia a few times. I travelled alone, but I wasn't always alone.

I was able to meet Francesca, my host sister from Milan who I lived with for six weeks on an exchange program I did at school in 2009. I also met Tommaso, an old ESL student of mine, in Milan. I stayed with my Australian friend, Lena, and her partner Pat in Germany. I also stayed with one of my past students, Albert, and his family in Germany, who made me feel like family, too.

I met Houssain in his new hometown, where I got some insight into his new life in Sweden.

I hired a car by myself and drove a fair way to go looking for seals! A seemingly insignificant achievement for most, but for me it was huge.

The last stop of my trip was Barcelona.

I studied Spanish there for a week. At the end of the trip, I met Annemarie, a fellow teacher from home, and we caught up for a few days before I returned home to Australia.

Why am I telling you all of this? It was so rewarding to travel alone and experience mental stability while doing so.

Organising my holiday, from flights, accommodation and all my side trips, gave me tremendous confidence that my trip would end perfectly.

My family and I had organised several plans, A, B and C, if my mental health was to deteriorate. I'm grateful we didn't have to enact any of those plans!

I also had friends and workmates, like Lozza, my high school friend, Emma, and my best workmate, Leticia, (not Dr Leticia) back in Australia who contacted me regularly to check in.

***

November 2019

Sarah

In November 2019, we picked Alice up from the airport after her trip to Europe. I was glad to have her back and so proud of her too.

Not everything went according to plan, but by having the options in place, she had a safety net. Alice was able to stand on her own two feet and come out on top.

Bravo, my darling, there is absolutely nothing you cannot do.

The journey that we have been on has shown us the depths of despair, the highs and the lows of life.

We have much to be thankful for and rejoice every day.

Open discussions with Alice allowed us more insight to her mental ill health. Thankfully, even while in the depths of psychosis, she allowed her doctors to share some of her journey with us.

Being open and compliant to taking her antipsychotic and antidepressant medications was of course a huge positive, especially early on in her recovery.

For Alice to be able to hear what we had to say and believe it over the voices in her head.

2020–2022

Alice

Since then, the COVID-19 pandemic hit.

I decided to stop working, teaching English and become a carer for my grandparents. I also picked up studying, choosing to study a Graduate Diploma of Psychology (GDP) online. Studying has been enjoyable but trying at times. I have learnt a lot and feel passionately about what I study, but it is a lot harder than my undergraduate degree was.

I have started working at a university as an ESL and academic adviser, part-time. At the end of 2022 I finished my GDP, and I am excited to commence my honours year in 2023.

I have also knocked an item off my bucket list, playing a season of Australian Football at a local club. I take my medication diligently, and I am always conscious of how much quality sleep I am getting. I am very open and honest about my condition, and I have friends who confide in me about their own mental health too.

I am confident in saying that I am an independent, strong person.

I am not obsessing over graduating from therapy, but instead I understand and accept that it may be a part of my life.

Sarah

We have all just started on this journey, who knows what it will hold or where it will lead. One thing I do know is that without her friends in Istanbul our girl would not be with us.

I have often thought, WHY has Alice done so well?

Why her?

The answer is I don't know.

What I can tell you is the first four years of Alice's mental ill health were extremely hard and an emotional roller coaster to say the least for all of us. Financially we took a hit, but that was the choice we made. I am well aware that many are not so fortunate. For Alice it was a time filled with psychotic thoughts, delusions, negativity, voices that echoed, anger and the verbal grenades that came our way. For Shane and me, it was often filled with sadness, uncertainty of what the future would hold and silence. Too afraid to paint Alice with the mental health brush and unwilling to *out* her. So, we remained silent.

We are mindful we walk on the edge. We will remain vigilant for triggers. Lack of sleep, alcohol, illicit drugs (we are blessed that Alice has not taken any since 2015) and lastly, bad relationships.

We celebrate Houssain and the other musketeers from Istanbul. Without them we would have had little to no chance of ever finding Alice. She would have been lost in 'the Bull' forever.

We rejoice in the dark tentacles being mostly gone.

Without the teamwork, love and support of Shane, Jess, Harry, Ella and our extended family and friends, our girl would not be where she is today.

Without the PECC unit in the public hospital, the USpace psychiatric unit and having Dr Leticia Aydos so readily available, she would be lost.

There is no old or new Alice, she is as wonderful as she has always been.

Alice is Alice.

But with her strength, her courage and her bravery, Alice can reach for the stars.

From *Dear Psychosis*,

I am strong.

I am proud.

I am ready to share.

I. Am. Breaking. The. Silence.

Epilogue

After writing this story, we all as a family thought that something was missing. We needed to write one last chapter. In no way am I telling you what to do in your own situations, these are just some of the times we did okay. Others where we did not. You may be able to add them to your own list or to ask a healthcare worker what they think.

To do this we need to go back to the beginning of our story and examine everything.

What we did well

The phone call
Houssain was clear and concise in his delivery over the phone and what he thought was happening to Alice.

What I did do well was bring Jesse into the equation, who was a calming influence, after I lost the plot.

Having a third person assist in those first few hours was necessary and extremely valuable as a second point of view. Jesse took control and steered the ship, asking the right questions to Alice's friends and being another set of ears listening to what Houssain was saying.

An extra helper

It was a brilliant call taking Jesse with me to Istanbul. I have no idea how I could have got Alice home if I was alone. This was only achievable because my parents stepped in. I am aware that not everyone has parents or friends or a credit card to help fund unexpected costs. We were indeed very fortunate.

I would advise, if at all possible, to have two people caring for your person dealing with psychosis, especially if you away from the home environment. Simple tasks like going to the toilet or waiting in queues can all be managed better if there are two of you. Of course, there will then also be two of you to chase after someone if they run. You will have one to mind the bags while the other two go to the bathroom. Most importantly, if you are travelling by bus, train or plane, there will be one extra person to stay awake and watch your person while the other sleeps.

Prior to leaving Australia

Before we left Australia, I did talk with a friend's father who is a psychiatrist for some advice. But as we were walking into the unknown of what was waiting for us, his answer was simple, get her home for evaluation and treatment if she needed it.

I also spoke with Beyond Blue and their advice was invaluable. I would never have thought to ring the Australian embassy for assistance.

Istanbul

The single most important thing was to get there.

Nearly-doctor Jesse taking a full medical history from Alice's friends was invaluable. You do not need to be a doctor to do this. Taking the time to go back in time with them to when they first all met, what she was like and when things started to change. What drugs if any were taken, what dosage and how many times.

The plane trip home

Having a plan of attack was necessary.

Getting to the airport early.

Being first in the queue.

Jesse's forward planning to clearing customs and thinking outside the box by going through the business class line. Although for us, this involved an abundance of luck.

Buying entry to a lounge. Sitting in the peace and quiet, able to eat, drink and go to the bathroom, without a plane load of people sitting around us.

Headphones

This may have been the single most brilliant idea that we completely lucked onto – Jesse giving Alice his headphones. Telling her if she didn't like a song to tap the button on the lead so it would skip a song and go to the next one. Alice called it 'nexting'. This meant when the voices overwhelmed her, she would do it and it would actually switch her brain for a second or two or three from the voices.

Locking and removing items

Fortunately, on the plane I was able to ask Shane to remove sharp objects at home, the paracetamol, ibuprofen, in fact anything that Alice could harm herself with. In Istanbul she made no mention of self-harm or taking medication to end her life but as a nurse it was one of my first thoughts. To remove any possible danger or harm, to take way temptation, to thwart the voices in her head if it became too much.

I don't think it matters where you put these objects, as long as it's not in a known hiding place.

What we could have done better

I wished that I could have been calmer when I received Houssain's phone call. Easy to say now.

I wish I had taken a carry-on bag only, rather than a suitcase. Why? Because all I needed was three days' worth of clothes. I could have washed undies and socks in the sink and there is no shame in wearing the same clothes for three days. In this case, less is more. Then you have less luggage to worry about handling, and you might even be able to skip having to wait at the luggage carousel at the airport.

Alice was hesitant to let anyone know that she was having delusions before she left on her trip. They were few and far between but enough to frighten her. She didn't tell us because she was scared. Then she rationalised it away in her head that it was just a little brain hiccup. The major factor I think was she thought her holiday might be cancelled.

Could we have checked in with more depth before she left? Could she have told someone?

The hardest thing to do is ask for help. There will be someone who will listen, a friend, a loved one, a helpline, doctor, nurse, teacher, your sports coach, a colleague. The most important thing to know is that you are not alone and you are loved. If you cannot say it aloud, write it on a piece of paper and give it to someone and say, 'I need your help'.

Breathe, my friend, breathe.

While she was away, I did ask her numerous times if she was ok but I suspect by the time I asked, Alice was already delusional so my questions came too late.

Home

Routine, routine, routine.

I wish I had implemented this as early as possible and been more mindful that Alice's life was completely out of control. The tentacles of psychosis were firmly knotted around her. She needed direction and consistency with everything.

The one thing we could control was a routine.

Getting up in the morning, breakfast, shower, five minutes of colouring in the adult colouring books, going for a walk, lunch, nanna nap, afternoon walk, prepare dinner, dinner, get ready for bed.

Day leave
Knowing that day leave was going to be a possibility, if I could do it over, I would get advice from the unit staff and then ensure that I had a plan of action. Our first day leave was a disaster. Think of somewhere quiet and peaceful, take a backpack with food, a rug, or chairs and decide whether you need to take another person with you. Especially if you are worried about being alone, you will all enjoy the day much better if none of you are stressed.

Feeling useful
What we forgot about was that Alice still wanted to feel needed and purposeful. We overlooked this until we went to Boomerang Beach on holidays and the café shop owner asked her to translate some information. Although it took her hours and no doubt caused anxiety, she felt amazing knowing that she was capable of doing something for someone else.

She felt appreciated.

Are you okay?
Asking the same question every day gets old, really fast.

There were two questions we would ask. 'How are you feeling?' and 'Are you okay?'

I wish we had implemented a simple colour-coded wrist band system. In the morning Alice could have put on the wristband that best described her mood.

Green – Calm

Orange – Ok

Blue – Anxious / depressed / voices
Red – High alert

We did not implement this as Alice was ambivalent about it. I think it would be a good way for our loved ones to express their mood without having to tell us. We could look at their wrist and immediately know what action to take. The band could be changed during the day, if things changed. Or some other colour-coded system that works for the individual. As a nurse I would love to do a simple study on this to see if it could be something that works.

Reading books, magazines, poetry ... anything
One of my biggest regrets is that I did not think of this earlier. What a calming way to bond and spend time with someone who is not well. You can literally read anything to them, poetry, magazines, novels, the list goes on. Alice would have loved this as long as it was not the news or something bad. It is seriously one of the simplest things to do and it is FREE.

What we learnt along the way

Family and friends support
My family knew but only my sister, one friend and my closest work colleagues 'really knew' of what was going on. So, for about the first twelve months after we got Alice home, we were silent and alone.

When we started talking to family and a small group of friends, I would always start the sentence with, "This is a cone of silence conversation." I was so anxious that Alice would be judged negatively for having drug-induced psychosis. I was dreading the questions of how, why, when, what, in fact anything.

We came up with a game plan and it was always the truth, honesty is the best policy.

Keep the facts short and sweet, yes, she is on medication, yes, she takes them. Most importantly I would always end with yes, we think she is amazing.

By coming up with a spiel, most of who we told were respectful of what we explained. Surprisingly, I would say more than half of those we told had either heard of a family member or friend going through something similar, or were themselves going through it. I have received phone calls after imparting our story from someone going through a mental health episode with one of their children. Asking for advice or simply wanting to talk to someone having been down the same path.

This is when I had my light bulb moment, thinking that we had something extremely special to share with others. With Alice's blessing, I became more confident about sharing our story to more than our select group of friends.

One of my wonderful friends, Janine, would ask me out for a cuppa. I would say 'no' and she said to me that she would never give up and she would keep asking me. I have not forgotten it and I will often use that phrase when I have had friends going through a hard time too. Keep the text messages going. All it needs is a smiley face, an offer to meet for coffee, a 'how are you today?' or 'I'm thinking of you.'

Alice's friends

This actually caused me no end of grief, watching friends slowly slip away. But you know what? It actually left a core group of the most amazing people that love Alice for her.

Forget about those that are fair-weather friends and focus on the ones that are there for the good and the bad.

Grief

It is ok to grieve what you have lost or feel out of control about.

The big question of, 'Will I ever get my son, daughter, loved one back?' is real.

Feeling anger, sadness, disappointment, and grief is OK.

Shoulda, woulda, couldas have no place now in my language.

What has happened is in the past. Looking back is helpful as long as we can learn from the experience.

Remember, this is a marathon, not a sprint.

None of us have a crystal ball.

Grieving for the life that your loved one once had is necessary. Let yourself do it, scream it out into the wind, let it blow away, do it every day if needed, who cares!!

Most importantly if you need to talk to a healthcare professional, please seek one out, they are the most amazing people and are out there waiting to support you.

Lastly

We were silent for way too long.

As a family we have decided to not only break that silence but to shatter it.

Perhaps it is fear that holds us back, but when the time is right, today, tomorrow, next year or in years to come, maybe one day, you too will join us.

Lastly, if we didn't share our experience.

The. Silence. Would. Continue.

Acknowledgements

WELL! Here I am now, having finished this most wonderful book.

I need to thank all those that have helped, supported and loved us along this journey.

To my amazing family, Shane, Jesse, Alice, Harry and Ella. Putting up with me tap, tap, tapping away, anywhere, and everywhere. Their never-ending support from the beginning, to celebrating the end. To my Har, for a young man to have such wisdom, strength and love shows that the world is your oyster and I cannot wait to see what the future holds. To Jess, thank you for showing me the way when I needed it the most, and for bring the beautiful Ella into our family. To my Shane, you have been my patience, my strength, my courage and my love since the day we first met and it has not dimmed.

I have had the most amazing support from my wonderful book buddies, we may have started out students together but you are now my dear friends. I met them through the Kelly Irving 'Expert Author Academy'. My best book buddy, the amazing Melissa Le Mesurier, who was up for all my weird questions and need for assurance no matter the time of day. Michelle Schiebner, Linda Garnett and Kelly Irving for all your encouragement and guidance to the end of the writing process.

To my sister Jane Fortini, who held my hand and was there for me whenever I needed her, again and again and never once complained. The best part was, she told anyone that would listen how proud she was of us.

To my beautiful mum and dad, Juju and Papa. You both are amazing and thank you for loving us all for just being us. To my brothers, David and Matthew, and their wonderful families who have encouraged us with love the entire journey.

To my wonderful friends, Shaunaugh, Scotty, Sharyn, Richard, Bruce, Darelle, Donna, Lindsay, Heidi M, Jacinta, Janine and Greg. My schoolie friends of over forty years Caroline Ch, Felicity, Gillian, Jacqui, Marea and Kelly, thanks for just being there for me. My wonderful mothers group, Anne, Robbie, Eliza and Sue, thanks for making me laugh and keeping me young. My Avondale golfing gals, who never minded me swearing on the golf course, Leesa, Caroline Cr, Ness, Jen, Mandy, Al, Rochelle, Sam, Jenny and Cath. This meant I was surrounded by love and support on some of the days I needed it most. All my work colleagues at NSSDH for all your love and support, Pip, Liz, Manny L and Manny M, Michael, Michelle, Simon, Georgia, Kerrie, Jenny, Elissa and everyone else, you may not be named but you are certainly not forgotten.

To my navy crowd. Shaunaugh and Scotty (yes, you get two mentions) Toddy, Nikki, James, Lynn, Bob, Michelle, Kylie and Robbo for your unfailing belief, love and support of our family and Alice's story.

To the wonderful group of readers who told it to me straight.

Houssain, Prof Gordon Parker, Dr Leticia Aydos, Heidi G, Caroline Cr, Greg and Chantal.

The editing, again, again and again, oh and the re editing, again and again. Thanks to the very talented editors extraordinaire, Lu Sexton and Stephanie Preston. I couldn't have done it without you fixing up my past, future and present! Yes, it was like that all muddled!!

To Dr Leticia Aydos, we could not have done it without you. We think you are an awesome person and a brilliant psychiatrist.

To my wonderfully talented friend Rebecca Hugonnet, for the cover design on the front and back. I cannot express my thanks enough.

A heartfelt thank you, goes to our Syrian crew, Rima, Kholod, Manar, Ba Sim, Basook and Batool.

Most importantly to Houssain. Without you, we would not have our Alice. Without a doubt you saved her from herself and the ravages of psychosis. Without you, we would have lost her. A mere thank you, my friend does not seem enough. We give you our heart and hope one day that we will meet again.

Lastly, but definitely not least, to my beautiful Alice, who is the bravest of all. To allow me the privilege to tell the world her story. To be able to describe her thoughts and feelings through her psychosis and bipolar illness was amazing in itself. To share this with others is such a selfless act that makes me the proudest mum of all. I love you my darling, YOU are amazing and I cannot wait to see what else the future holds for you.

To all that have read our story, a heartfelt thank you and

please remember you are not alone.

If we do not speak out about mental ill health, the silence will continue.

#talk

Further resources

Australia

Please call 000 in an emergency

Beyond Blue
beyondblue.org.au

Black Dog Institute
blackdoginstitute.org.au

SANE Australia
www.sane.org

Head Space Australia
headspace.org.au

The Man Cave
themancave.life

Mental Health Australia – Emerging Minds
emergingminds.com.au

Mental Health and Suicide Prevention
health.gov.au/health-topics/mental-health-and-suicide-prevention

New Zealand

health.govt.nz/your-health/services-and-support/health-care-services/mental-health-services

USA

nami.org

UK

mentalhealth.org.uk

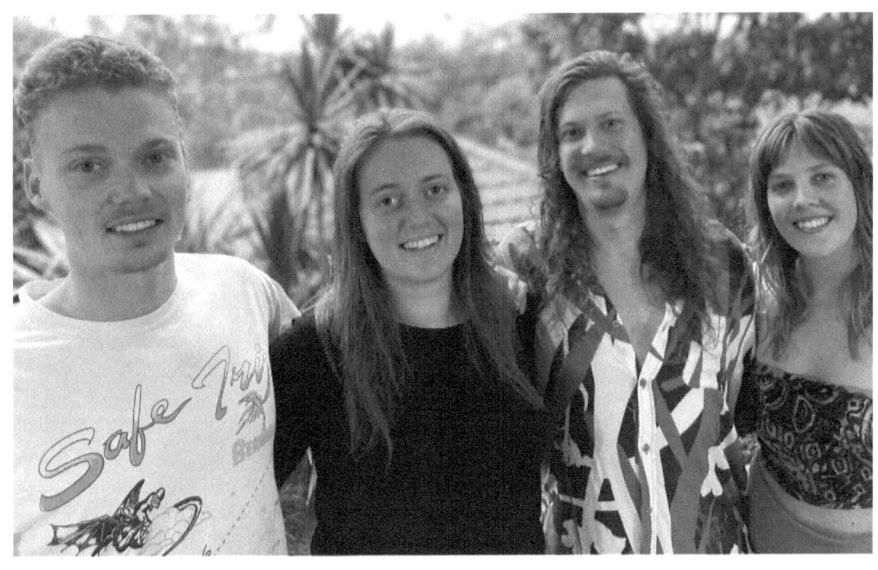

Left to right: Harry, Alice, Jesse & Ella, Christmas 2022

www.ingramcontent.com/pod-product-compliance
Lightning Source LLC
Chambersburg PA
CBHW030254010526
44107CB00053B/1702